# PAIN MANAGEMENT: DON'T FORGET NUTRITION

## WILLIAM ACKERMAN MD

PAIN MANAGEMENT:  DON'T FORGET NUTRITION

Copyright © 2016 by WILLIAM ACKERMAN MD

I wish to dedicate this book to my significant other for her support while I wrote this book and who insists that I adhere to proper nutrition as well as exercise in spite of how busy I am.

# Acknowledgments

I would like to extend my thanks to my patients with chronic painful conditions who complied with changing their dietary habits as well as initiating exercise programs and decreasing their medications to reduce their overall chronic pain.

# Table of Contents

1. PAIN OVERVIEW ........................................................................ 1

2. PAIN CAUSITION ...................................................................... 7

3. PAIN TREATMENTS ................................................................. 15

4. COST OF TREATMENT ............................................................ 19

5. PAIN ASSESSMENT ................................................................. 25

6. PAIN DOCTOR CREDENTIALS ............................................... 31

7. DIAGNOSTIC TESTS ............................................................... 35

8. ADDICTIVE DRUGS ................................................................ 41

9. ADDICTION ............................................................................. 49

10. ACUTE PAIN .......................................................................... 53

11. ANTIINFLAMMATORY MEDICATIONS ................................. 59

12. MUSCLE RELAXANTS ........................................................... 66

13. ANTICONVULSANTS ............................................................. 75

14. ANTIDEPRESSANTS .............................................................. 81

15. TOPICAL AGENTS ................................................................. 87

16. ALTERNATIVE THERAPIES .................................................. 97

17. CHIROPRACTIC THERAPY .................................................. 107

18. BEHAVORIAL TERAPY ......................................................... 111

19. PHYSICAL THERAPY ............................................................ 117

20. NECK PAIN ........................................................................... 125

21. BACK PAIN ........................................................................... 133

22. MUSCLE PAIN ...................................................................... 145

23. FIBROMYALGIA ................................................................... 151

24. HEADACHES ........................................................................ 157

25. NEUROPATHY........................................................ 167

26. OSTEOPOROSIS ..................................................... 175

27. JOINT PAIN............................................................ 181

28. SHINGLES ............................................................. 191

29. REFLEX SYMPATHETIC DYSTROPHY ..................... 199

30. SPORTS PAIN......................................................... 207

31. HIV ....................................................................... 215

32. CANCER ................................................................ 221

33. VASCULAR............................................................ 233

34. CHEST PAIN .......................................................... 241

35. ABDOMINAL PAIN .................................................. 249

36. BEHAVORIAL PAIN.................................................. 259

37. ELDERLY PAIN ....................................................... 265

38. PALLATIVE CARE ................................................... 271

39. HOSPITALIZED PATIENT ......................................... 275

40. NUTRITIONAL CONSIDERATIONS ............................ 279

# 1. PAIN OVERVIEW

Almost everyone experiences pain at some time. Pain can be a natural response to injury and disease in some instances. With the advent of pain medicine as a medical specialty, patients no longer need to suffer. Suffering is how our lives are affected. Patients who suffer have significant reductions in the normal joys of their lives. They cannot enjoy their families or enjoy recreational activities etc. Their pain affects them emotionally.

Pain is an unpleasant sensory and emotional experience following tissue injury. Pain occurs as a response to tissue irritation, injury, infection, ischemia or inflammation. Surgery may help decrease tissue irritation if it is caused by a disc herniation etc. Antibiotics may stop pain caused by infections. Injury treatment may require steroids, orthopedic surgery, chiropractic, physical therapy etc. Ischemia may require surgery or a stint. Inflammation may decreased by a proper diet such as the Mediterranean diet. The Mediterranean diet emphasizes eating foods like fish, fruits, vegetables, beans, high-fiber breads and whole grains, nuts, and olive oil. Meat, cheese, and sweets are very limited.

Most pain however is a result of inflammation. Nutrition may be therefore helpful in decreasing inflammatory pain. Patients should try to avoid strong narcotic medications for any type of pain. Anti-inflammatory medications, anticonvulsants, steroid injections and mild pain medications may be of benefit. This book in addition to conventional pain management addresses nutrition for pain reduction. Unfortunately, it is the rare physician who includes diet therapy and nutritional supplements in patient care.

Pain is a complex, idiosyncratic experience. When pain is the primary complaint for seeking medical attention, understanding of multiple factors is essential in guiding successful treatment. Behavioral medicine, a branch of psychology, has been an integral part of interdisciplinary/multidisciplinary care of pain patients. Prominent and distressing emotions, cognitions, and behaviors frequently accompany chronic pain. In many cases, these psychological symptoms will be sufficiently severe to qualify the patient for a diagnosis of a mental disorder.

Chronic pain is a disease. Your doctor will strive to provide you with a quality of life. If your pain is acute such as post-surgical pain, or after a fall on your hip you should expect significant pain relief. Chronic pain is that pain that persists after your body has healed. Nothing unfortunately will completely eliminate your pain.

The goal of pain management is to decrease your pain so that you can maintain your normal activities of daily living. This means that your pain should not interfere with your work, family or recreation. As a result, if you have chronic pain your goal and your doctor's goal should be to decrease your pain to a tolerable level.

Because many pain treatments will not benefit you, it is necessary for you to become an informed consumer. You can do this by trying to understand what is causing your pain and what alternative modalities (such as chiropractic, herbs etc.) are available to you. If you complain of pain to your primary care physician, your doctor may refer you to someone who only treats pain.

According to a recent Institute of Medicine Report on Pain, 100 million Americans suffer from pain. Treatment of pain costs the United States more than half a trillion dollars per year. Pain is one of the most common reasons people consult a physician. Yet it frequently is inappropriately treated.

Americans spend over one hundred billion dollars annually on pain care. One-third of all adult Americans suffer from chronic pain. Over the counter annual analgesic cost of medical care is rapidly escalating. Employers may not be able to afford health insurance for their employees. The cost of pain management is contributing to the increase in health care costs and amounts to hundreds of thousands of dollars. As a result, there is considerable profit to be made by unethical health care providers that include hospitals as well as physicians.

The specialty of pain management enables many individuals with chronic pain to improve their quality of life. Patients who are unable to pay however are frequently excluded from treatment. You should also be aware that the American Board of Medical Specialties has a list of specialties recognized as true medical specialties or subspecialties in the United States. Pain management itself is not included in this list.

However, the American Board of Anesthesiology added qualification in pain medicine is recognized. Physicians other than anesthesiologists such as physical medicine and rehabilitation, neurologists etc. can become board certified. This should tell you "Buyer beware!" Many patients use the Internet to access information regarding pain management. In my practice, less than ten percent of patients obtain medical information from an academic source such as the National Library of Congress from computer sources.

This book will enable you to gain a basic knowledge of the pathophysiology (the cause of your pain) and the treatment of various nutritional entities which may reduce your pain. This will enable you to become a team member with your doctor. This knowledge should help prevent you from becoming a potential victim by avoiding the incompetence of certain physicians who claim to be "pain medicine specialists" and by avoiding procedures that are possibly dangerous or have absolutely no scientific merit.

The pharmaceutical perspective of inflammation focuses on relieving symptoms through over-the-counter analgesics and far more powerful prescription drugs. There is a need however, to address the nutritional influences on chronic inflammation as a means of decreasing some painful symptoms.

Health care professionals should query patients about their nutritional intake, recognizing that adjustments in the types of foods consumed can often address long-standing symptoms that create distress, including pain, fatigue, anxiety, and gastrointestinal dysfunction.[1]

Inflammation is one of the causes of chronic pain and this can be related to diet. The ratio between omega six and omega-3 fatty acid's used to be 1 to 1 to 2 to 1 in the average diet twenty years ago. Today it is 20 to 30 to 1 in the Average American diet. This causes chronic inflammation. Trans fatty acids in the diet are bad they can inhibit the formation of enzymes that are needed to decrease the inflammatory process.

Pro-inflammatory chemicals include linoleic acid, vegetable (oil corn and saffron oil), and arachidonic acid. These are free radicals and cause inflammation and pain as well. Many of the inflammation-sustaining fats are found in common cooking oils and packaged foods.

When a balance of dietary fats is restored, through diet and supplements, the body regains its natural ability to both turn on and turn off inflammation. Elevated blood sugar (glucose) levels, stemming from a diet with too many refined carbohydrates and sugars, also can increase inflammation in the body. People with insulin resistance commonly have high levels of C-reactive protein, a sign of inflammation. Insulin resistance is at the heart of Syndrome X and type 2 diabetes. Syndrome X, which increases the risk of both diabetes and heart disease, is also marked by fat around the waist, high blood pressure, and high cholesterol and triglycerides.

Given that no two people are alike, if you are taking any medications and begin to take nutritional supplements you should be aware that potential drug-nutrient interactions may occur and are encouraged to consult a health care professional before using any natural product. Combining certain prescription drugs and dietary supplements can lead to undesirable effects such as: diminished prescription drug effectiveness, reduced supplement effectiveness and impaired drug and/or supplement absorption.

The American diet contains chemicals which cause inflammation. Processed foods cause inflammation. The immune system regulates inflammation. Chemical that cause inflammation include: omega 6 fatty acids (vegetable oils such as corn, safflower, peanut, cottonseed, and soy oils, as well as in processed and packaged foods containing these oils), trans fatty acids (salad dressings, breakfast bars, shortening, nondairy creamers, stick margarines, and many baked items such as cakes and cookies), and free radicals which are hazardous molecules that damage the body's cells.

Antioxidant nutrients help control inflammation. The oniega-3 family of fatty acids supplies powerful anti-inflammatory substances. The parent fat of the omega-3s, alpha-linolenic acid, is found in dark green leafy vegetables and flaxseed. Antioxidants such as vitamins E and C are nutrients that neutralize free radicals. Linoleic acid is the basis of all the other omega-6 fatty acids. Too much of it causes chronic inflammation. The widespread use of vegetable cooking oils-in kitchens, restaurants, and packaged foods-is a reason for the prevalence of inflammatory disorders.

Your body converts linoleic acid to more powerful compounds like arachidonic acid, which is converted into eicosanoids. Eicosanoids include such substances as prostaglandin E. The conversion of arachidonic acid is then converted to substances such as prostaglandin E. Other pro-inflammatory compounds include proteins called cytokines. Some of these cytokines, such as interleukin-6 leukin-6 and C-reactive protein cause the formation of many pro-inflammatory compounds.

If your diet is dominated by linoleic acid your body will make large amounts of inflammatory causing compounds. Diets rich in olive oil reduce the severity of inflammatory disease such as rheumatoid arthritis. The vast quantity of omega-6 fatty acids in the American diet encourages chronic inflammation.

Free radicals are found in virtually all unsafe chemicals, including air pollutants and cigarette smoke, and are generated when your body is exposed to radiation. Free radicals stimulate inflammation. The natural remedies for free radicals are antioxidants, which include vitamins E and C and many other nutrients. The many flavonoids found in vegetables, fruits, and herbs directly counteract the pro-inflammatory effects of free radicals.

Vitamins, minerals, proteins, and fats-are the building blocks of your entire body. They form not only your skeleton, skin, and organs, but are also the basis of your hormones and the multitudes of biochemicals involved in forming new cells and tissue, healing injuries, and creating energy. For example, a recently published study on the beneficial components of white mulberry leaves exhibiting their biological activity in the various pathological and health human ailments.[2] Pomegranates alleviate disease activity and improves some biomarkers of inflammation and oxidative stress in rheumatoid arthritis patients.[3]

The vast majority of dietary carbohydrates and calories come from highly refined grains such as wheat, corn and rye, and sugars (sucrose and high-fructose corn syrup, in soft drinks and other beverages, and fried potatoes. Many individuals are allergic to gluten, causing what is known as celiac disease. In these people, eating gluten triggers an inflammatory response, which primarily attacks tacks the gastrointestinal tract and interferes with vitamin and mineral absorption.

Gluten sensitivity may appear as immunological reactions affecting the nervous system, balance, and behavior, as well as a person's overall sense of well-being. Lectins play a role in rheumatoid arthritis and possibly other inflammatory autoimmune diseases.

A reader of this book must remember that there is never a "one size fits all "approach to pain management. Each patient must be evaluated and treated on an individual basis after the cause of the pain has been identified. Remember that trauma pain and ischemia may require surgery, pain related to infection may require antibiotic therapy, and irritation related pain may require steroid injections at the site of the irritation and inflammation may require anti-inflammatory medications.  Proper nutrition may be overall effective in pain reduction as well.

References

1.       Sandquist L. Food First: Nutrition as the Foundation for Health. Creat Nurs. 2015;21(4):213-221.

2.       Gryn-Rynko A, Bazylak G, Olszewska-Slonina D. New potential phytotherapeutics obtained from white mulberry (Morus alba L.) leaves. Biomed Pharmacother. 2016;84:628-636.

3.       Ghavipour M, Sotoudeh G, Tavakoli E, Mowla K, Hasanzadeh J, Mazloom Z. Pomegranate extract alleviates disease activity and some blood biomarkers of inflammation and oxidative stress in Rheumatoid Arthritis patients. Eur J Clin Nutr. 2016.

# 2. PAIN CAUSITION

Pain is caused by an injury to a nerve ending. The injury can be caused by inflammation, injury, ischemia (lack of blood flow), irritation or infection. Pain impulses are in essence, electrical signals that travel from various areas of your body such as the extremities, heart, appendix etc. to the spinal cord and eventually reach the brain where the pain signals are processed like data in a computer. The brain is like a computer hard drive, which stores painful experiences that ultimately results in the suffering associated with chronic pain.

Pain is produced by unpleasant stimuli to nerve endings throughout the body which include chemical, extreme heat cold and mechanical injury. These nerve endings are silent until mechanical, heat or cold injures tissue. In order to experience pain we need these pain receptors and the nerve fibers that transmit pain to the spinal cord and then to the brain.

Nerves, which conduct pain impulses to the spinal cord, are composed of neurons (nerve cells) that make up nerve fibers that form neurons. Two common pain fibers are the C fibers and the A-delta fibers. A-delta fibers conduct fast onset sharp pain impulses. The C fibers conduct slow onset dull, aching or burning pain. If you hit your finger with a hammer, you will experience a sudden pain response followed by a dull pain response.

Other types of fibers that transmit touch and vibration exist do not cause pain in most instances. However, these fibers can become hypersensitive and may contribute to your total pain experience. A neuron is an electrically excitable cell in the nervous system that processes and transmits information. Neurons are the significant core components of your brain and spinal cord as well as your peripheral nerves.

Neurons are typically composed of a cell body, a dendrite and an axon. Neurons receive input from denrites and transmit output via the axon. Neurons are the building blocks of nerves. In other words, multitudes of neurons are necessary to form a nerve. Nerves that exist outside of your central nervous system are called a ganglion.

Your stellate ganglion in your neck is an example. An injection into this ganglion may relieve pain associated with Reflex Sympathetic Dystrophy (now called Complex Regional Pain Syndrome). Various ganglia may form a plexus. An example of a plexus is your celiac plexus. Sometimes this plexus is blocked with numbing medicine, phenol or alcohol to relieve severe abdominal pain.

Dendrites

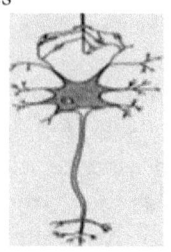

Axon

Figure 1. A nerve is composed of neurons. A neuron has one axon that takes nerve signals away from the neuron. The long end of the axon communicates with multiple dendrites.

Action potentials generated by the neuron initiate pain signals. If your skin is pinched a mechanical pain receptor begins and action potential. An action potential begins after a depolarization (a change in the electrical activity within the neuron) such that it could cause a membrane transitory modification, turning prevalently permeable to sodium ions more than to potassiu ions. Sodium permeability can cause an action potential.

Neuropathy generates a local accumulation of sodium channels, with a consequent increase of density. This remodel seems to be the basis of neurohyperexcitability. Calcium channels have also an important role in cell function. Intra-cellular calcium increase contributes to depolarization processes, through kinase and determines the phosphorylation of membrane proteins that can make powerful the efficacy of the channels them-selves.

Following an acute injury, AMPA receptors are stimulated which cause sharp pain. Receptors (areas in the body where biochemicals or drugs attach) are present in the spinal cord are called NMDA (N-methyl-D-aspartate) receptors and cause chronic pain. When these NMDA receptors are stimulated, pain becomes more severe and this severe pain is maintained which implies that the pain does not decrease. The brain is responsible for the suffering associated with pain. Pain results in bodily responses especially with respect to the cardiovascular system (heart rate increases, blood pres-sure increases, renal arteries constrict etc.).

When pain is severe, the brain can cause the body to increase both the heart rate and blood pressure. Severe pain can also result in profuse sweating as well as nausea and vomiting. There are different types of nerve endings throughout the body. The pain nerve endings become hyper excitable when stimulated by injury, inflammation or a tumor. Occasionally the nerve endings re-main irritable even after the painful stimulus has been removed.    Pain signals from areas in the body reach the brain by four processes (transduction, transmission, modulation and perception).

Axons carry pain fibers away from your neuron and direct them to the dendrites of the next neuron until they terminate in your brain or spinal cord.  Remember that the axons and dendrites do not touch.  They form synapses or clefts between the axon and dendrite.  The synapse has chemicals in the axon nerve ending.  These chemicals allow communication between the neurons.  Drugs are chemicals that can interrupt the communication between the neurons.  Hypnosis and biofeedback can disrupt pain signal transmission.  Injections can also inhibit transmission of pain signals from your arms or legs to your brain.

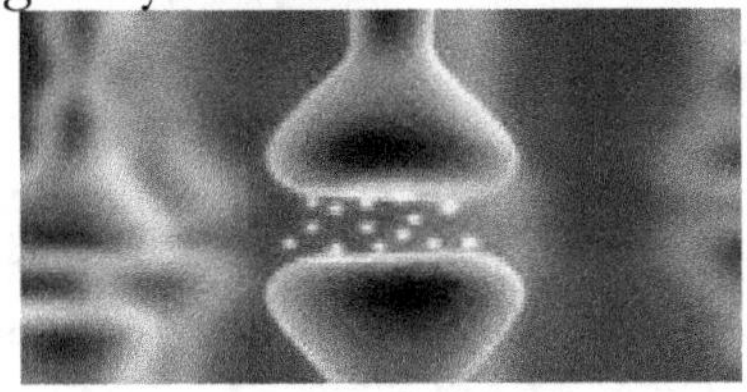

Figure 2.  Chemicals are transferred between nerve endings (synapses) which cause transmission of pain signals. Pain signals may be blocked if the chemicals are inhibited from passing from one nerve to another.

You need to understand that pain signals cross to the opposite side from the injury and therefore travel to the opposite side of your brain. Figure 3 demonstrates this concept.  The following illustration demonstrates by the arrows that pain signals enter the back of your spinal cord.  They cross over to the other side. The pain impulses will then proceed upwards to go to your brain.  It is important to know that pain signals can be dampened by structures and chemicals that exist in your spinal cord. Pain signals as mentioned previously are trans-mitted from the site of injury as action potentials. Electrical and/or chemical activity between the neuron dendrites and axons propagate the axon potentials. Pain signals enter your spinal cord, then cross to the other side of your spinal cord and proceed upward to your brain. Pain on your right side goes to the left side of your brain.

It is important to understand the following processes in order to under-stand how your pain can be treated effectively.  Transduction is a process where electrical signals originate in the nerve endings throughout your body. These impulses are chemically, mechanically and/or thermally mediated and transmitted to your spinal cord where they can be modulated and then sent to your brain. Tissue injury or disease (including arthritis) cause the body to release biochemicals called prostaglandins. Prostaglandins themselves do not cause pain.  Prostaglandins do however sensitize pain receptors to other chemicals in the body, which facilitate the trans-mission of pain impulses. Nonsteroidal drugs like ibuprofen decrease the number of prostaglandins produced in your body and may in a decrease in your pain perception. Topical creams such as Ben Gay can decrease the process of transduction at the nerve endings.

Transmission is a process where pain signals are transported to the spinal cord. Nerves in body tissues transmit impulses to the spinal cord. Nerve blocks with anesthetics like Novocain can interrupt the transmission of pain impulses to the spinal cord. Once pain impulses reach the spinal cord they are modulated or changed by chemicals and nerves that inhibit or lessen the number of pain impulses from going up the spinal cord to your brain. Fibers called internuncial fibers are present within the spinal cord that can decrease pain transmission.

The brain can send impulses back to these pain control fibers within the spinal cord to decrease the number of impulses that reach the pain perception center of the brain. This is the basis of hypnosis. Severe pain however, over-whelms the nerve fibers and hypnosis essentially becomes ineffective. Most pain impulses cross over into the opposite side of the spinal cord from where they entered the spinal cord.

The spinal cord acts like a transformer to intensify or decrease the intensity of pain impulses. Narcotics and anticonvulsants can modulate pain impulses within the spinal cord. Finally, pain impulses reach the brain where you perceive pain. Be aware that pain signals enter the posterior part of your spinal cord and then cross to the other side and travel upwards to the pain processing of your brain.

Narcotics can "numb" your brain to decrease the effects of the pain impulses on your brain by decreasing the intensity of these impulses. Higher brain centers determine how we respond to a painful stimulus. This explains why an individual can respond differently to a painful stimulus from other individuals (e.g. "cry baby, whiner, vs. macho man etc.). A chapter describing the anatomy and physiology of pain is not complete without an explanation of the Gate Control Theory of pain.

Melzak and Wall described this theory in 1965. Different types of nerve fibers (both pain and non-pain fibers) enter the spinal cord at the same time. Non-pain fibers essentially dilute out the number of pain impulses that enter the spinal cord. An example of the Gate Control Theory is given by the following analogy.

If you can imagine severe pain impulses represented by of multiple black balls going down a sink (analogy to spinal cord). If one adds multiple white balls (neutral non-pain transmitting entities), the number of black balls (pain impulses) is diluted. Therefore less severe pain impulses reach the spinal cord and the brain. The white balls are non-pain balls and can close the gate (drain) to the number of black balls that go down the sink. To open the gate to more pain impulses, one only needs to decrease the number of white balls going to the hole in the sink. At this time, there are more black balls (pain impulses) available. The gate is now open.

As you can see, pain perception in the human body is complex. Because there are many different chemical transmitters and anatomic structures that contribute to chronic pain syndromes, each patient's treatment must be individualized. This is where the art of pain medicine is separated from pure science.

In order to understand pain transmission concepts, you must first become familiar with several biochemicals that are stored in your body that affect your pain signals. In order for you to hurt, pain-producing chemicals in your body tissue must stimulate pain fibers (Alpha-delta and C fibers). In general, the greater the tissue trauma, the more pain transmitting chemicals are produced and the worse the pain.

In medical terminology, a stimulus (pin prick) produces a response (pain perception). When a stimulus such as heat produces, tissue injury chemicals are released at the site of nerve injury, which cause pain fibers to become hyperactive. These chemicals include bradykinin, histamine, substance p, acetylcholine, serotonin and histamine. These chemicals act at the nerve endings and ultimately travel to the spinal cord and brain.

The nerves that conduct pain go to the spinal cord that allows pain signals to ultimately reach the brain. Areas of your body that have many pain receptors include the skin, the outer aspect of bone called the periosteum, ligaments, joints, teeth and gums and the cornea of the eye.

Muscle also contains pain fibers but not as many per square meter (a measure of area) as the previously mentioned structures. Where the nerves from your body enter your spinal cord, aspartic and glutamic acid are produced. These acids increase pain impulse generation.

NMDA may also be produced. GABA (gamma-aminobutyric acid) in the spinal cord on the other hand, decreases the number of pain impulses that reach the brain. GABA inhibits pain impulse transmission. Norepinepherine and serotonin are two more chemicals in the spinal cord which attenuate the number of pain impulses which reach your brain. The brain and spinal cord regulate pain by the production of naturally occurring narcotic-like substances that decrease pain transmission in specific areas of the brain. These narcotic-like drugs are called enkephalins, dynorphins and beta-endorphins. Some of these substances also decrease pain transmission in the spinal cord. Enkephalins are located in areas of the brain related to pain modulation.

Enkephalins inhibit pain at the spinal cord level. Enkephalins bind to narcotic receptors. When the narcotic receptors are activated, they inhibit pain signals. Dynorphins exist in both the brain and spinal cord but are more prevalent in the brain. Like enkephalins these substances bind to narcotic receptors in the brain and spinal cord.

Pain impulses that enter your spinal cord cross over to the other side and then progress upward to your brain. The natural beta-endorphins in your body exhibit morphine-like activity. They work like morphine to decrease your pain. Following injury or stress these endorphins are released into the blood stream.

The effects of beta-endorphins are similar to morphine. Beta-endorphins like narcotics can cause respiratory depression, constipation, euphoria, toler-ance and physical dependence. The exact biochemical actions of all of the sub-stances mentioned are complex. For a more de-tailed explanation of the actions of these substances one should consult a pain medicine text-book. The purpose of this chapter is to emphasize the multiple substances that can generate the transmission of pain signals.

This is furthermore the reason why there are so many medications available for the management of your pain. This is also the reason why your physician may prescribe multiple medications for the management of your chronic pain. The injury causes transduction of the nerve ending which means that the nerve ending is stimulated to begin sending pain impulses to your brain where you perceive the pain.

Transmission of the pain impulses sends pain signals to the spinal cord where pain signals are modulated and then are sent to the brain. Inflammation can cause transduction of your nerve endings which ultimately causes your pain experience.

Almost everyone experiences pain at some time. Pain can be a natural response to injury and disease in some instances. With the advent of pain medicine as a medical specialty, patients no longer need to suffer. Suffering is how our lives are affected. Patients who suffer have significant reductions in the normal joys of their lives. They cannot enjoy their families or enjoy recreational activities etc. Their pain affects them emotionally.

Pain is an unpleasant sensory and emotional experience following tissue injury. Pain is a complex, idiosyncratic experience. When pain is the primary complaint for seeking medical attention, understanding of multiple factors is essential in guiding successful treatment. Behavioral medicine, a branch of psychology, has been an integral part of interdisciplinary/multidisciplinary care of pain patients. Prominent and distressing emotions, cognitions, and behaviors frequently accompany chronic pain. In many cases, these psychological symptoms will be sufficiently severe to qualify the patient for a diagnosis of a mental disorder.

Chronic pain is a disease. Your doctor will strive to provide you with a quality of life. If your pain is acute such as post-surgical pain, or after a fall on your hip you should expect significant pain relief. Chronic pain is that pain that persists after your body has healed. Nothing unfortunately will completely eliminate your pain.

The goal of pain management is to decrease your pain so that you can maintain your normal activities of daily living. This means that your pain should not interfere with your work, family or recreation. As a result, if you have chronic pain your goal and your doctor's goal should be to decrease your pain to a tolerable level. However, is some instances, nutrition to decrease pain is seldom addressed.

Chronic inflammation can cause pain and is a sign that something has gone seriously askew with your health. Instead of protecting and healing your body, chronic inflammation breaks down your body. It may ultimately be a result of your nutritional habits which in turn causes your pain.

Certain nutrients help form your body's inflammation-promoting compounds, which normally help fight pain impulse conduction. Others help produce your body's anti-inflammatory substances, which moderate and turn off inflammation which subsequently decreases or stops the pain.

Omega-3 and omega-6 fatty acids are precursors of bioactive lipid mediators posited to modulate both physical pain and psychological distress.

Because inflammation causes pain, a reduction in your pain could possibly occur with proper nutrition. There are studies which suggest that some dietetic elements (polyunsaturated fatty acids, Mediterranean diet and antioxidants) have anti-inflammatory effects and may decrease inflammation.[1]

Reference

1.      Gonzalez Cernadas L, Rodriguez-Romero B, Carballo-Costa L. [Importance of nutritional treatment in the inflammatory process of rheumatoid arthritis patients; a review]. Nutr Hosp. 2014;29(2):237-245.

# 3. PAIN TREATMENTS

This chapter presents a general overview of modalities available to treat your pain. The ability to relieve pain is very variable and unpredictable, depending on the source or location of pain and whether it is acute or chronic. Pain mechanisms are complex and have peripheral and central nervous system aspects. Therapies should be tailored to the specifics of the pain process or processes in the individual patient.

Anesthesiologists do nerve blocks and prescribe narcotic medications. Physical therapists will rehabilitate your body. Chiropractors manipulate your spine to control your back and neck pain by realigning your spine and taking pressure off your nerves.

Surgeons operate on nerves, joints and discs to lessen the suffering of pain. In many chronic pain states a multidisciplinary approach using all or most of the mentioned pain specialists is used to manage complex pain problems such as reflex sympathetic dystrophy which will be described in a later chapter.

Which modalities actually work? Each of these modalities can help you with your pain. In many instances a multidisciplinary pain center can provide you with the most benefit. You should investigate what therapies are scientifically sound. You should have some basic knowledge about scientific studies that have been.

Nerve blocks are frequently used to manage pain. Local anesthetics like Novocain used in combination with steroids are deposited near the nerves or tissues that are responsible for chronic pain. These anesthetics stop pain production by numbing the nerves responsible for your pain. The steroids decrease the irritability of the pain producing nerves. In many instances these blocks will break the pain cycle.

Many patients respond to drug therapy. Mild and strong narcotics are prescribed depending on the severity of your pain. Pain patches with either a local anesthetic or a strong narcotic exist which give a patient sustained pain relief. Long acting narcotics (Oxycontin) exist which decrease the need for frequent drug dosing.

Antidepressants and anticonvulsants modulate pain transmission in the spinal cord. Muscle relaxants decrease muscle spasm that can significantly decrease your pain. Non-steroidal anti-inflammatory drugs alleviate pain by decreasing tissue inflammation. The Chinese have used acupuncture for over 2000 years. This method of pain relief consists of placing small needles into the skin and muscles over the body. The needles stimulate larger nerves that go to the spinal cord and release endorphins and enkephalins. These substances decrease the number of pain impulses that go to the brain. Chiropractic therapy consists of manipulating the spine by a physician trained in safe spinal manipulation.

A chiropractor aligns the spine. This maneuver takes pressure off the nerves coming off the spinal cord that decreases pain conduction. Psychologists may help control pain with hypnosis or biofeedback. Hypnosis helps activate the nerves in the spinal cord that block pain signals from traveling up your spinal cord to your brain. Biofeedback uses a machine to enable a pain patient to relax painful muscle.

Physical therapists administer modalities that provide heat and cold to your muscles and ligaments. Some therapists do massage therapy that relaxes painful muscles. Electrical stimulation applied to the body decreases pain in a variety of painful conditions. The device is called a TENS (Transcutaneous Electrical Nerve Stimulator) unit. This instrument is battery powered.

A TENS unit stimulates endorphin and enkephalin production in your spinal cord. Neurosurgeons can place implantable devices in your body to control severe pain. One device is called a narcotic pump. This device gives a drop of morphine or other strong narcotic into the fluid around the spinal cord.

The other surgically implanted device is called a spinal dorsal column stimulator. A wire is attached to a battery source that is placed in your body. The wire is placed parallel to your spinal cord. This stimulation releases endorphins and enkephalins within the spinal cord. As one can see many modalities are available to patients for the control of their chronic pain.

Given that no two people are alike, if you are taking any medications and begin to take nutritional supplements you should be aware that potential drug-nutrient interactions may occur and are encouraged to consult a health care professional before using any natural product. Combining certain prescription drugs and dietary supplements can lead to undesirable effects such as: diminished prescription drug effectiveness, reduced supplement effectiveness and impaired drug and/or supplement absorption.

Which one is right for you? The proper treatment for your pain will depend on the severity of your pain as well as your physical and mental health status. Be aware that the pathogenesis of joint diseases are for the most part unknown, a number of nutrient and non-nutrient components of food have been shown to affect the inflammatory process and, in particular, to influence clinical disease progression. For example, the action through which the Mediterranean diet pattern exerts its beneficial effects on patients remains to be elucidated, but it has been shown that arthritis patients may potentially benefit from it in view of their increased cardiovascular risk and the treatment they require which may have serious side effects.1

This book will present nutrition as another means to help decrease a patient's pain. Be aware however that drugs, surgery etc. can potentially have serious side effects. the pathogenesis of joint diseases are for the most part unknown, a number of nutrient and non-nutrient components of food have been shown to affect the inflammatory process and, in particular, to influence clinical disease progression and cause pain.

Reference

1.     Oliviero F, Spinella P, Fiocco U, Ramonda R, Sfriso P, Punzi L. How the Mediterranean diet and some of its components modulate inflammatory pathways in arthritis. Swiss Med Wkly. 2015;145:w14190.

# 4. COST OF TREATMENT

Approximately forty-eight million Americans suffer from chronic pain. According to a previous Wall Street article, Americans spend over 100 billion dollars on pain care. Over one third of all adult Americans suffer from chronic pain. Over the counter annual analgesic costs amount to three billion dollars. Chronic pain is a prevalent and a costly problem. One must assess the clinical effectiveness and cost-effectiveness of the most common treatments for patients with chronic pain.

Untreated or under treated chronic pain costs health plans and their purchasers a lot of money. It afflicts 40 million or more Americans, with a cost of nearly $100 billion a year in direct medical costs and indirect costs, such as lost productivity and workers' compensation, according to the American Pain Society. Chronic pain with conservative care such as medications, physical therapy, chiropractic etc. costs North American adults an estimated $10,000 to $15,000 per person per year.

After rapid growth during the 1980s and through the mid-1990s, the number of inpatient chronic pain management programs actually declined. Concurrent with the decline in intensive programs is the rise of procedural interventions and medications, which receive a great deal of support from hospitals and pharmaceutical companies. The use of muscle relaxants for patients appears to be increasingly prevalent when compared with teaching relaxation techniques, and implanting a device is more lucrative than giving patient's guidance or advice.

Healthcare specialists have to determine whether this apparent shift in treatment emphasis away from rehabilitation is a healthy development for the patients they serve. Many hospitals encourage physicians with minimal or no training to open pain clinics in their facilities. They can charge facility fees of $1000.00 or more for a procedure like an epidural steroid injection. Your physician doing the procedure may own shares in the center or hospital. As a result, every time that a physician schedules a procedure in the hospital he or she makes a share of the profit. The sad fact is that this behavior is legal.

Medical procedures, such as trigger-point injections, sympathetic nerve blocks, and epidural steroid injections, are rated as significantly less helpful, less invasive modalities; despite their considerably higher average cost. The cost of chronic benign (non-cancer pain) spinal pain is large and is increasing. The costs of interventional treatment for spinal pain were at a minimum of $13 billion (U.S. dollars) in 1990, and the costs are growing at least 7% per year.

The interventional medical treatment of chronic pain costs $9000 to $19,000 per person per year. It should be understood that only a small percentage of patients receive long-term relief with these procedures. You should inquire about the cost of any treatment before agreeing to have the procedure done. You also need to contact your insurance carrier and ascertain if your treatment is covered under your insurance plan.

Your treatment for your back pain may only cost $3.00 for a bottle of aspirin. However, you need to calculate and add your chiropractor fees or the costs of a massage. What about the housekeeper you had to hire to do the housework that you can't do while you were disabled? What about the heating pad? What does it cost you if you need to cut down on the hours you work, or quit your job because of your pain? Pain costs can affect your family if your spouse has to take off work to help you.

Pain treatment can be expensive for you but a question arises concern-ing the cost of you not receiving pain management. Pain patients frequently miss work because their pain is too severe to allow them to work. As a result business productivity can be decreased. Lost work-days also cost businesses money. The overall cost of pain amounts to over sixty billion dollars per year.

You need to ascertain if you have to pay co-payments and how much those costs are. You also need to know whether the balance of the charge beyond the co-payment will be billed to your insurer, or whether you have to pay in full when the service is provided and then request reimbursement from your insurer. You should also ask your insurance company if it will pay for alternative medicine therapies like acupuncture.

If you could look at your past 12 months and calculate how much time that you lost from work because of your pain and compare these figures to your cost of receiving care, you can estimate the actual cost of your treatment. For example, if an epidural steroid injection costs $500.00 but saves you 3 days of lost work time at $200.00/day, you actually save $100.00. If an injection keeps your activities of daily living normal, then one would expect the treatment to be cost effective if the treatment itself is effective.

Professional fees charged by physicians may differ from doctor to doctor. In some areas of the United States, physicians will post their professional service fees somewhere in their office so that you are informed of the costs before you consent to a procedure. Before you seek medical care, you should call several pain management offices to ascertain professional fees. Your primary care physician will then refer you to a physician that you chose.

In the United States, chronic pain is often poorly treated at an exceedingly high cost. Consultation costs were a significant proportion of cumulative healthcare cost. Health economists from Johns Hopkins University writing in The Journal of Pain reported the annual cost of chronic pain is as high as $635 billion a year, which is more than the yearly costs for cancer, heart disease and diabetes. Results showed that mean health care expenditures for adults were $4,475.

Estimates for pain conditions were 10 percent for moderate pain, 11 percent for severe pain, 33 percent for joint pain, 25 percent for arthritis, and 12 percent for functional disability. Chronic pain is pain that lasts more than several months (variously defined as 3 to 6 months, and is longer than normal healing. It's a very common problem.

Persons with moderate pain had health care expenditures $4,516 higher than someone with no pain, and individuals with severe pain had costs $3,210 higher than those with moderate pain. Similar differences were found for other pain conditions: $4,048 higher for joint pain, $5,838 for arthritis, and $9,680 for functional disabilities. Also, adults with pain reported missing more days from work than people without pain. Pain negatively impacted three components of productivity: work days missed, number of annual hours worked and hourly wages.

Opioids are widely accepted as treatment for moderate to severe pain, and opioid-induced constipation is one of the most common side effects of opioids. Patients using opioids with newly diagnosed constipation had significantly greater healthcare utilization and costs than patients without constipation.as published in a study by Fernandez et. al in 2016. These costs accounted for approximately 16% of the total healthcare costs per patient during the 12-month study period. Recognition and effective treatment of opioid-induced constipation may decrease healthcare utilization for patients with chronic noncancerous pain and may reduce the economic burden of pain therapy.

Economic arguments are not sufficient to accept substitution of generic medications in musculoskeletal disorders. Low back pain in general and specifically chronic low back pain forms a major burden for the patient and society. Recently studies demonstrated that up to 65% of patients evolve to chronic pain in the study published by Itz et. al in 2016. The process of trial and error of different specialties and treatment possibilities often results in a long and costly trajectory. A better understanding of the subtypes of chronic low back pain, the risks for chronification and fast adequate referral may result in higher patient satisfaction and cost reduction.

Sacroiliac joint (SIJ) disorders are common in patients with chronic lower back pain. Minimally invasive surgical options have been shown to be effective for the treatment of chronic SIJ dysfunction. Compared to traditional non-surgical treatments, SIJ fusion is a cost-effective, and, in the long term, cost-saving strategy for the treatment of SIJ dysfunction due to degenerative sacroiliitis or SIJ disruption.

The low costs of local anesthetics, the small number of consultations needed, the reduced intake of analgesics, and the lack of adverse effects also suggest the practicality and cost-effectiveness of this kind of treatment. The application of local anesthetics alone durably improves pain symptoms in referred patients with chronic and refractory pain. The low costs of local anesthetics, the small number of consultations needed, the reduced intake of analgesics, and the lack of adverse effects also suggest the practicality and cost-effectiveness of this kind of treatment.

Physical therapy was more common with chronic pain or obesity comorbidities and less likely to primary care entry; physical therapy entry was associated with lower 1-year costs. Although few patients entered care in physical therapy, this modality may be useful for managing costs.

Relative to acute pain, which lasts for a short time, chronic pain can persist for years. It can be triggered by an injury or infection, or cancer, but can occur without of bodily damage. Common complaints include migraines, back pain and arthritis pain. Most patients will usually undergo a lengthy process of trial and error before finding the right treatment. The costs of chronic pain emotionally and financially, personally and societally are too high to ignore.

Given that no two people are alike, if you are taking any medications and begin to take nutritional supplements you should be aware that potential drug-nutrient interactions may occur and are encouraged to consult a health care professional before using any natural product. Combining certain prescription drugs and dietary supplements can lead to undesirable effects such as: diminished prescription drug effectiveness, reduced supplement effectiveness and impaired drug and/or supplement absorption.

A program has been developed for chronic pain sufferers, primarily those with low back and cervical spine pain. The treatment is a six-week interdisciplinary program including relaxation training, gradually increasing exercise, and significant education on behavioral and exercise strategies and nutrition for long-term pain management. This program is inexpensive, cost efficient, and may be implemented easily in a variety of settings.[1]

There is literature that supports the idea in which the Western diet and inactivity are proinflammatory whereas a plant-based diet and activity are anti-inflammatory. Lifestyle behavior change can be integrated into osteoarthritis management through teamwork and targeted evidence-based interventions. Healthy living can therefore be exploited to reduce inflammation, oxidative stress, and related pain and disability and improve patients' overall health.[2]

Eicosanoids are major players in the pathogenesis of several common diseases, with either overproduction or imbalance often leading to worsening of disease symptoms. It is known that there are interactions between diet and drugs in the pathogenesis and therapy of various common diseases.

A high omega-6/omega-3 fatty acid concentration ratio in meat, and eggs (because the omega-6/omega-3 ratio of the animal diet is unnaturally high) directly leads to exacerbation of pain conditions, cardiovascular disease and most cancers. The health economic benefits of such products for society as a whole must be anticipated to outweigh the direct costs for the farming sector.[3] Nutrition support is indeed a cost-effective therapy that benefits patients.

References

1.      Wells MJ, Peay A. Interdisciplinary Treatment of Musculoskeletal Pain: The EMPOWER Program. J Back Musculoskelet Rehabil. 1993;3(1):54-63.

2.      Dean E, Gormsen Hansen R. Prescribing optimal nutrition and physical activity as "first-line" interventions for best practice management of chronic low-grade inflammation associated with osteoarthritis: evidence synthesis. Arthritis. 2012;2012:560634.

3.      Christophersen OA, Haug A. Animal products, diseases and drugs: a plea for better integration between agricultural sciences, human nutrition and human pharmacology. Lipids Health Dis. 2011;10:16.

# 5. PAIN ASSESSMENT

Pain is a subjective experience for which there are no objective biological markers. There is no objective measurement of pain. Self-report is considered the most accurate and appropriate pain assessment method as family members and caregivers often underestimate a patient's pain. Pain is a complex entity and is affected by tissue injury but also by previous pain experiences, as well as by your psyche (anxiety and depression) and by any pending lawsuits.

The transition from acute pain following an injury to chronic pain cannot be explained. The entity that we refer to as pain cannot be touched or felt by the treating physician. As a result, you must give your doctor an accurate assessment of your pain. Many chronic pain patients have seen a variety of physicians before seeing a pain medicine specialist. Many patients become frustrated and sometimes feel that no one believes that they truly hurt.

A patient's pain may not correlate with findings or lack of findings on a physical examination and X-rays. A patient's pain can only be adequately diagnosed after the treating physician has done a good history and physical examination. A clinician cannot feel your pain. As a result, you will be given papers to fill out with questions to answer. Questions asked will include a history of your pain, a pain diagram and occasionally a depression and/or activity assessment. Significant depression can worsen your pain.

Several different techniques are available for your doctor to use in determining your level of pain. Commonly used techniques include verbal, visual, and psychological tests. Both you and your doctor are responsible for documenting and recording trends in the intensity and frequency of your pain. This information tells each of you whether your pain has really improved or whether it has worsened.

Charting your pain levels in a diary will help your doctor see your long-range (weeks-months) pain trends, which are ultimately more important than your day-to-day pain trends. One important factor used to assess your progress is your activity. Also your daily diet needs to be assesses to identify foods which may cause inflammation as well as pain.

Your doctor will depend on you for accurate and reliable answers to questions about the pain you experience. Because pain involves many aspects such as sensory, emotional, and behavioral factors, it is difficult to measure the amount of pain you feel based on one single parameter. The choice of a pain-assessment test depends on the needs of both you and your doctor.

For example, if you just complain of a toothache, your doctor will have almost no way of knowing how severe your pain condition is. There is no general consensus among pain medicine doctors as to the best test for the measurement of pain. An ideal test for the assessment of pain must bring together experimental as well as clinical knowledge.

One way of assessing your pain is to use a numeric scale. This is the simplest method for attempting to measure your pain. During this test, you are asked to rate your pain on a scale of 0 to 5 or to use words such as "none," "slight," "moderate," or "severe." This assessment is also a quick, simple, and reliable way to evaluate the effectiveness of any medications you are taking to manage your pain.

On the numeric scale, 0 equals no pain, 1 equals mild pain, 2 equals moderate pain, 3 equals distressing pain, 4 equals horrible pain, and 5 equals excruciating pain confining you to bed rest. This method is easily understood and may be helpful in guiding the treatment plans your doctor creates for you. Another type of verbal scale asks you to rate your pain on a scale of 1 to 10, with 1 being equivalent to pain that is barely noticeable and 10 relating to excruciating pain. A verbal numeric scale is easily understood. All you have to do is choose a number to represent your level of pain.

Another method used by some doctors is a pain diary. This is a descriptive report you keep to assess your pain. The pain diary shows a written account of your day-to-day experiences. It can be used to help diagnose the causes of your pain. The value of the pain diary is that you and your doctor can monitor your day-to-day variation of painful states and your response to therapy. You need to keep a diary of your pain patterns when you are sitting, standing, and lying down. You should also record your sleep patterns and sexual activity. You also must note the amount of pain medication you are taking and whether it lessens your pain. Because pain can interfere with eating patterns, keep a diary of the amount of food you eat and at what time you ate. Be sure to include any types of recreational activities and whether your pain felt better or worse afterward.

Pain drawings offer a visual way to evaluate your pain. You will be asked to shade in areas on a human figure outline that correspond to the areas of your pain. The drawing will help your doctor determine where your pain is coming from and how widespread it is on your body. Over time, your pain drawings can be compared to show the changes of your pain and how you are responding to therapy.

After observing your behavior, your doctor may classify your pain behavior by using the following four-class system: Class 1 consists of patients with low physical injury but high levels of abnormal behavior patterns related to their pain. Class 2 consists of patients with lower physical injury and low behavior pattern abnormalities. Class 3 consists of patients with significant tissue injury in addition to high behavioral pattern abnormalities. Class 4 consists of patients with a high tissue injury and normal behavioral patterns.

A McGill pain questionnaire is a method for assessing pain psychologically. A McGill pain questionnaire gives a multidimensional pain score. You are given 20 word sets that describe a different dimension of your pain. You are asked to select words relevant to your pain from each of these 20 sets. For example, one set includes the words "jumping," "flashing," and "shooting." Another set includes the words "tingling," "itching," "smarting," and "stinging." You circle the word that relates closest to the pain you feel throughout the 20 word sets.

The McGill pain questionnaire consists of four different parts. The first part consists of a human figure drawing on which you are instructed to mark the location of your pain. The second part is the pain-rating index that contains 78 words divided into 20 groups. Each set contains up to six words. Five of these groups describe tension or fear. Each word is assigned a value according to its position within a subclass. The third part of this test asks additional questions about prior pain experiences, as well as the location of your pain and current usage of pain medications. The fourth part consists of a present pain intensity index. This aspect of the test requests a pain score from 0 to 5 with word descriptors such as no pain, mild pain, discomforting pain, distressing pain, or horrible and excruciating pain. These words also are assigned different values. All the values are added to obtain a total score. All the scores are then evaluated to attempt to assess your total pain experience.

There is also a short form of this test that has been developed. This questionnaire contains fewer words and categories than the long form. This test is sensitive to evaluations of reduction in pain experiences. This test is more useful for rapid evaluation of data following procedures or surgery.

Other pain self-assessment scales are available. The horizontal visual analog scale consists of a 10 cm line anchored by two extremes of pain: no pain and extreme pain. Patients are asked to position a sliding vertical marker to indicate the level of pain they are currently experiencing; pain severity is measured as the distance in centimeters between the zero position and the marked spot. The vertical visual analog scale is similar to the prior scale but is presented vertically, and the line is replaced by a red triangle with its summit facing downwards (no pain=0) and its base at the top (maximum pain=10). The faces pain scale consists of a line drawing of seven faces that express increasing pain (no pain=0, maximum pain=6.

Many pain physicians use Verbal Analogue Scales (VAS) to assess the severity of your pain. A scale of 0 to 10 can be used. A score of 0 indicates no pain while a score of 10 represents the worst imaginable pain. This scale is simple and is easy to be understood by the patient. This is similar to the previous scale with the exception that a patient makes a mark on a ruler with marks from 0 to 10. Your pain ratings will be kept in your patient chart and the scores will be compared with each visit. These scales serve as a gauge of your progress to treatment.

Some doctors want to have their patients keep a pain score diary on a daily basis. Your doctor may want to know the relationship between your pain and your activity such as sitting, standing and walking. Since sleep deprivation can worsen your pain, your doctor may ask you about your sleep pattern on each visit. Your doctor needs to know if you can do normal activities as well as whether or not you can work. In order for a physician to formulate your treatment plan, your physician needs to know if the pain is localized or referred. Localized pain is confined to one area such as a knee joint.

Referred pain begins in one area and travels to other areas of your body. An example is pain referred from the heart during a heart attack to the left arm. A pain medicine specialist also needs to know if your pain is superficial or deep. An example of superficial pain is that from a fingernail or from the skin as seen following sunburn. An example of deep pain is that from a structure deep within the body such as a diseased appendix or gallbladder. One treatment may only require medications while the other may require surgery. As you can see the treatment for each of these types of pain will differ. Superficial pain may be treated by analgesic creams or by pills.

Deep pain as seen in cancer patients may require needle injections or surgery to control the pain. Referred pain such as pain originating from the heart may require a surgical procedure or may require only medications. Localized pain can be treated with an injection of anesthetics that can numb the painful area. An example is an injection of a knee joint. You should begin to understand that the treatment of pain could be complex and on occasion be frustrating for both the patient and physician.

Before a physician begins pain treatments, a complete examination must be done. Strength, sensation and reflexes must be evaluated. Skin temperature should be noted as well as range of motion of the neck, back and extremities. A patient's mental status must be evaluated. Vital signs and the way a patient walks should be recorded. Swelling, skin color and hair loss should be appreciated. Loss of sensation to touch can be evaluated by rubbing a fine brush over the skin. Strength and coordination are evaluated as part of the neurological examination. Following your examination your physician will probably want to order diagnostic studies. Plain X rays are used to diagnose bone abnormalities of the spine. A CAT scan is used to define bone abnormalities, as well in more detail than a plain X ray.

You may ask why your doctor cannot diagnose the source of your pain by looking at your laboratory or imaging studies. These studies only relate that there is an abnormality in your pathology. You need to know that if you have abnormal tests, it does not mean that you hurt. If you have degenerative disc disease noted on X ray, you do not have to have pain. The X-ray is only a picture. For example, you may have a picture of a telephone. Is it ringing? There is no way to tell from looking at the picture that you are in pain. The same is true with respect to imaging studies and laboratory tests.

An MRI is useful for the diagnosis of soft tissue pathology such as nerve compression or muscle shrinkage, disc herniations and tumors. However, the MRI does not tell if you hurt. You can have a disc herniation, but not experience any pain. A myelogram is the injection of dye into the fluid that surrounds the spinal cord. This test can visualize a disc herniation or compression of a nerve coming off of the spinal cord. A bone scan is the injection of dye into your vein followed by a series of pictures of your skeleton that are recorded by a scanner. This test can detect arthritis and trauma to bone as well as tumors. An EMG is the evaluation of your muscle using needle electrodes. This test can detect muscle pathology.

Nerve conduction studies evaluate abnormalities of the transmission of electrical impulses through nerves. Blood tests can detect rheumatoid arthritis and some medical diseases such as liver disease. A urinalysis may detect kidney pathology. As you can see the diagnosis and treatment of chronic pain can be difficult and challenging. Because pain can have multiple causes, a physician must treat you as a whole and not just your area of pain. For example, you may have pain in the bottom of your feet. This pain may be the result of a vitamin deficiency. Your doctor could give you some numbing medicine (e.g. a Lidoderm patch) for your feet that may decrease your pain for a short time. However, if your vitamin deficiency is corrected, your pain may completely resolve.

The verbal rating scale is a simple, commonly used pain rating scale. To complete it, subjects select one of six descriptors that represent pain of progressive intensity: none, mild, discomforting, distressing, horrible, or excruciating. Another scale is a modified 21-point Box Scale. The scale has a row of 21 boxes labeled from 0 to 100 in increments of five. The 0 is labeled "no pain," while the 100 score is labeled "pain as bad as it could be."

Pain can be extremely difficult to assess in elderly patients. It can be difficult for elderly patients to give a numeric representation of their pain. They should be asked to verbally describe their pain as none, some or severe. Pain may be particularly difficult to identify in cognitively impaired individuals as it can manifest itself atypically as agitation, increased confusion, and decreased mobility. In many clinical settings, pain is not assessed in demented patients due to reliability concerns. In particular, self-assessment is rarely attempted. Furthermore, when pain is evaluated in severely demented patients, the nursing staff routinely uses observational scales. These assessments include vocalizations, facial expressions, and body language.

Pain is also difficult to diagnose in infants and children. Children less than two years of age will report that they hurt but have difficulty localizing the exact area where they hurt. A child with a finger injury may just report pain but not identify the finger as the source of pain. This is because the brain has not developed enough to be able to distinguish generalized pain from localized pain. As a result infants and young children must be observed. Crying, facial expression and blood pressure and heart rate can be good indicators that pain is present.

If you have inflammation in a part of your body then extra protein is often released from the site of inflammation and circulates in the bloodstream. The erythrocyte sedimentation rate (ESR) and C-reactive protein (CRP) tests are commonly used to detect the increase in protein. In this way they are used as markers of inflammation. The CRP test measures the level of one specific protein, whereas the ESR takes account of many proteins.

# 6. PAIN DOCTOR CREDENTIALS

Doctors who manage pain are frequently anesthesiologists. Anesthesiologists ensure that you are safe, pain-free and comfortable during and immediately following surgery. But not everyone realizes that decades of research and work done by anesthesiologists have led to the development of newer, more effective treatments for patients who have pain unrelated to surgery. Many techniques used to make surgery and childbirth virtually painless is now being used to relieve other types of pain. In fact, the work pioneered by anesthesiologists has led to treatments for pain control outside the operating room.

Frequently an anesthesiologist heads a team of other specialists and doctors who work together to help you manage your pain. Pain medicine doctors are experts at diagnosing why you are having pain as well as treating the pain itself. Some of the more common pain problems they manage include: arthritis, back and neck pain, cancer pain, nerve pain, migraine headaches, shingles, phantom limb pain for amputees and pain caused by AIDS. Pain medicine doctors are experts at diagnosing why you are having pain as well as treating your pain.

Like other physicians, anesthesiologists have completed four years of medical school. They spent four more years learning anesthesiology and pain medicine during residency training. Many anesthesiologists who specialize in pain medicine receive an additional year of fellow-ship training to become an expert in treating pain. Some also have done research, and many have special certification in pain medicine through the American Board of Anesthesiology. This board is the only organization recognized by the American Board of Medical Specialties to offer special credentials in pain medicine. Medical specialty certification in the United States is a voluntary process. While medical licensure sets the minimum competency requirements to diagnose and treat patients, it is not specialty specific. Board certification demonstrates a physician's expertise in a particular specialty and/or subspecialty of medical practice. Pain medicine is a subspecialty of anesthesiology.

The American Board of Medical Specialties member boards (24) are responsible for setting the standards for quality practice in a particular medical specialty. Each Member Board has a board of trustees or directors, all of whom are certified in that Board's medical specialty. Individual Member Boards evaluate physician candidates to ascertain if the candidate completed the appropriate residency requirements and if he or she has an institutional or valid license to practice medicine. If a physician meets these basic admission standards, the Member Board will evaluate the candidate using written and oral examinations. Because specialties differ so widely, the criteria that inform these tests are quite different. What makes someone a good anesthesiologist does not necessarily make him or her a competent cardiologist.

Ultimately, the measure of physician specialists is not merely that they have been certified, but that they keep current in their specialty. The American Board of Medical Specialties requires maintenance of certification that is a formal means of measuring a physician's continued competency in his or her certified specialty and/or subspecialty. To become recertified a physician must: hold a valid, unrestricted medical license, meet educational and self-assessment programs determined by the particular Board, demonstrate specialty-specific skills and knowledge, demonstrate the use of best evidence and practices compared to peers and national benchmarks. Specialists in Physical Medicine and Rehabilitation are eligible to take the pain management specialty boards as well.

Unfortunately, a physician needs no credentials to practice pain management other than a medical or osteopathic medicine degree and a state medical license. As a result, there are no guidelines as to who can call themselves a pain medicine "specialist". There are no local, state or national standards with respect to pain management. The American Academy of Pain Medicine, the American Academy of Pain Management, and the American Board of Anesthesiologists administer written examinations to certify pain management doctors. These organizations provide continuing education courses annually. Some physicians do not certify through one of these organizations but classify themselves as pain physicians. They may go to a weekend cadaver course to be able to do a certain procedure.

Ask to see your physician's credentials. Hospitals in many instances may want anyone who will show up and has a medical degree to do potentially mutilating procedures on patients who have insurance. You should ascertain if your pain doctor has completed a fellowship (specialized training in pain medicine) or has sufficient experience through residency training to do a procedure on you. With these facts in mind, you must do your homework when choosing a pain medicine physician. Most university pain centers require that pain medicine physicians have a formal fellowship before they can begin to treat patients.

It is your duty to find the best-trained physician. Your insurance plan will list doctors approved by their plan. Some companies have strict criteria before admitting physicians to their plan. A physician should have some certification from a medical specialty like anesthesiology, physical medicine etc. to do pain medicine in addition to completion of a fellowship. Ideally, the pain medicine physician should have further training in pain medicine.

If your physician has no certification in any specialty you should eliminate that physician from your list of potential treating physicians. There may be some qualified doctors who have not taken a certification test but it would be extremely difficult identifying those individuals who are truly competent. You should ask your physician if he or she has credentials in pain medicine including research publications etc. To ascertain if your physician is certified by the American Board of Medical Specialties, go to the website www.ABMS.org.

# 7. DIAGNOSTIC TESTS

Information obtained from laboratory tests may help doctors decide whether other tests or procedures are needed to make a diagnosis of your health. The information may also help your doctor develop or revise a patient's treatment plan. All laboratory tests are generally used along with other exams or test such as MRIs, X-rays, and EMGs etc.

The doctor who is familiar with their patient's medical history and current condition is in the best position to order and to explain test results and their implications. Patients are encouraged to discuss questions or concerns about laboratory test results with the doctor. Two common tests that you should be familiar with are the complete blood count and the blood chemistry tests.

A complete blood count measures the levels of different types of blood cells. By determining if there are too many or not enough of each blood cell type, a CBC can help to detect a wide variety of illnesses or signs of infection. A blood chemistry test measures the levels of certain electrolytes, such as sodium and potassium, in your blood. A C reactive protein and erythrocyte sedimentation rate teat may be useful in the diagnosis of rheumatoid arthritis or other inflammatory diseases.[1]

Doctors order urine tests to make sure that your kidneys are functioning properly or when they suspect an infection in your kidneys or bladder. This is important if you are taking a medication like a nonsteroidal anti-inflammatory medication that can affect your kidney. A urine test can be done in the doctor's office or even at home. It's easy for toilet-trained kids to give a urine sample since they can urinate in a cup. In other cases a catheter (a narrow, soft tube) can be inserted through the urinary tract opening into the bladder to get the urine sample.

Tylenol (acetaminophen) can cause liver damage if you take too much (more than 4000 mg per day). Liver function tests ascertain how your liver is working and helps diagnose any sort liver damage or inflammation. Your doctor may order one when looking for signs of a viral infection or liver damage from other health problems. On occasion, blood tests may be done to determine that you do not have a bleeding problem such as hemophilia. Aspirin can cause bleeding by decreasing the ability of your blood to clot. Before doing a nerve block it is prudent to know if your blood will clot in a normal time. Otherwise a needle can result in significant bleeding.

Plain X rays can be done in a physician's office. X rays can assess bone-joint arthritis. X rays can diagnose degeneration of your discs. Your bone alignment (do the bones line up with each other?) can be assessed as well. Bone fractures can also be identified. You should be aware that you are subject to radiation exposure with this diagnostic test. If you have the possibility of having osteoporosis, your physician may order a DEXA (dual energy x-ray absorptiometry) that is a specific test for the diagnosis of osteoporosis. A Computed Tomography (CT scan) allows a physician to assess a disc in your back as well as arthritic changes affecting the bones in your neck and back.

A CT scan of your head can also be useful for the diagnosis of a bleeding injury to your brain following trauma to your head. Patients receive radiation exposure with this test. Myelography or a myelogram is primarily of use when surgical therapy is planned. A dye is placed in the fluid that surrounds your spinal cord. An image is formed which tells a physician that a nerve coming off your spinal cord is compressed or not compressed by a disc herniation.

An image does identify painful areas of your body. An image only demonstrates abnormal anatomy that could be an area of pain generation. Degenerative disc disease noted on an X- ray for example does not imply that you have a disease or are supposed to have pain. This entity is a normal aspect of aging. Therefore, you should not be alarmed if your doctor tells you that you have degenerative disc disease. The same is true if you are told that you have a disc herniation. Not every disc herniation causes pain and not every disc herniation requires surgery.

Ultrasound is another valuable diagnostic tool. Though ultrasound tests are typically associated with pregnancy, doctors order ultrasounds for different reasons. For example, an ultrasound test can be used to look for collections of fluid in your body, or for problems with your kidneys.

Computerized axial tomography is a specialized x ray. CAT scans are a kind of X-ray, and typically are ordered to examine for pathologies such as appendicitis, internal bleeding, or abnormal organ growths. The technique is used in diagnostic studies of internal bodily structures, as in the detection of tumors or brain aneurysms. A scan is not painful.

Generally a CT is preferred where bone details necessary (long bones like your arm or leg, spine, skull), while a MRI produces much better soft tissue details (brain, spinal cord etc.) CT scans are useful for examining body cavities (thorax, abdomen, pelvis) for calcium deposits, cysts, and abscesses.

Magnetic Resonance Imaging (MRI) is done by utilization of a magnetic field that is applied around your body. MRIs use radio waves and magnetic fields to produce an image. MRI's (Figure 2) are often used to look at bones, joints, and the brain. Contrast material is sometimes given through an IV in order to get a better picture of certain structures. The MRI involves no radiation.

A MRI cannot be done if you have certain metals in your body or a heart pacemaker or a defibrillator. Magnetic resonance imaging allows visualization of the discs, spinal cord and cerebrospinal fluid. A MRI can be used with a contrast dye to identify an extruded disc, infection or tumor.

Plain X rays give physicians images in a front to back plane. A side-to-side plane and an oblique view are helpful in diagnosing possible causes of your pain. On the other hand, a CT and MRI image shows slices of the body as well as a three hundred and sixty degree image of a defined section of the body.

Images only show pathology. They do not show pain. Pain is a subjective experience. If you view a photograph of an old scratched and dented telephone, you have no idea if it is ringing or not. You have no idea if it works. The same is true with an X- ray image. An abnormal X ray does not mean that you hurt.

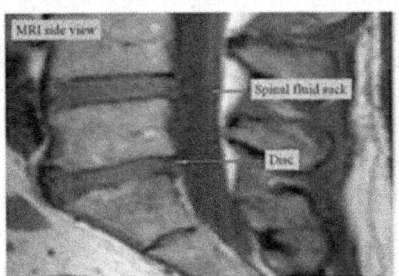

Figure 1. MRI from a side view. Note that when compared to a plain X ray that you can see more anatomic structures.

Bone scanning is done using a technetium isotope tracer injected into a vein. This tracer is distributed according to the bone blood flow. A greater blood flow to the bone from trauma such as a fracture or arthritis is compatible with greater bone absorption of the tracer. Total body radiation occurs but is low following a bone scan.

The three-phase bone scan consists of the administration of a radioactive tracer followed by scanned images on three occasions. The first image is phase 1 Phase one measures blood flow on the first pass of the tracer. The second phase assesses the blood vessel system while the third phase assesses the turnover of bone, which can be seen in fractures or tumors. Bone scans are frequently used to diagnose RSD.

Electromyography (EMG) and the Nerve Conduction Velocity tests (NCV) are two diagnostic tools that are helpful to the pain management doctor. These two tests allow the assessment of the location, the pathogenesis, and the prognosis of neuromuscular lesions.

A NCV measures how fast your nerve sends and impulse. Stimulation of the nerve is done at one end of your nerve and the velocity is measured at another end of your nerve. Generalized nerve pathology results in a reduced nerve conduction velocity. In other words your nerve impulses are slower than normal.

Electromyography (EMG) measures the response of muscles and nerves to electrical activity. It's used to help determine muscle conditions that might be causing muscle weakness, including muscular dystrophy and nerve disorders. A needle electrode is inserted into your muscle (the insertion might feel similar to a pinch) and the signal from the muscle is transmitted from the electrode through a wire to a receiver/amplifier, which is connected to a device that displays readout. EMGs can be uncomfortable and scary to kids, but aren't usually painful. Occasionally kids are sedated while they're done.

Distal latency is the assessment of the distal conduction velocity of your painful nerve that can be affected by the neuromuscular junction that is the location where the nerve and muscle join. Some muscle diseases may have normal NCV studies but electromyographic (EMG) abnormalities usually occur in these situations. EMG measures muscle electrical activity.

The NCV assesses the speed at which your peripheral nerves transmit electrical signals. Your nerve is stimulated, usually with surface electrodes, which are patch-like electrodes placed on your skin over the nerve at various locations. One electrode stimulates the nerve with a very mild electrical impulse. The other electrode records the resulting electrical activity. The distance between electrodes and the time it takes for electrical impulses to travel between electrodes are used to calculate the nerve conduction velocity.

A normal muscle should contract when stimulated by a nerve impulse. A needle electrode is inserted through the skin into your muscle. There should be a short burst of electrical activity at this time. The electrical activity detected by this electrode is displayed on an oscilloscope, and may be heard through a speaker. After placement of the electrodes, you may be asked to contract certain muscles. The presence, size, and shape of the waveform make up an action potential. This waveform provides information about the ability of your muscle to respond to electrical stimulation.

These tests are useful for investigating nerve and muscle function in diseases such as peripheral neuropathy, compression neuropathy etc.

Reference

1.        Jack Challem. The Inflammation Syndrome: The Complete Nutritional Program to Prevent and Reverse Heart Disease, Arthritis, Diabetes, Allergies, and Asthma (Kindle Location 199). Kindle Edition.

# 8. ADDICTIVE DRUGS

Narcotic drugs are prescribed for postoperative pain, cancer pain and for some chronic pain syndromes. Narcotic drugs can relieve moderate to severe pain. The term narcotic refers to agents that benumb or deaden nerves, causing loss of feeling or paralysis. Psychodelic drugs like LSD, contrary to popular belief are not narcotics. Many law enforcement officials in the United States inaccurately use the word "narcotic" to refer to any illegal drug or any unlawfully possessed drug.

Most medical professionals prefer the term opioid which refers to natural, semi-synthetic and synthetic substances that behave pharmacologically like morphine. The Opioids are a class of controlled pain-management drugs that contain natural or synthetic chemicals based on morphine, the active component of opium. These narcotics effectively mimic the pain-relieving chemicals that the body produces naturally. Opioids are the most often prescribed pain-relievers because they are so effective.

Morphine is the standard to which other opioid drugs are compared. Morphine is frequently prescribed to alleviate severe pain after surgery. Codeine can be helpful in soothing somewhat milder pain, as are oxycodone (OxyContin, an oral, controlled-release form of the drug), propoxyphene (Darvon), hydrocodone (Vicodin), hydromorphone (Dilaudid) and meperidine (Demerol), which is used less often because of its side effects. Dipheoxylate or Lomotil can also relieve severe diarrhea, and codeine can ease severe coughs.

The primary medical use of opioids is to relieve pain. Other medical uses include control of coughs and diarrhea, and the treatment of addiction to other opioids. Opioids can produce euphoria, making them prone to abuse. Opioids should only be used for moderate to severe pain that has not responded to non-narcotic drugs like aspirin or ibuprofen.

Narcotics can be used alone like oxycodone or used in combination with aspirin, ibuprofen or acetaminophen (Tylenol). Some narcotics like oxycodone or morphine are available as an extended release tablet that must be swallowed whole. Tablets, which are not extended release, may be split..

In 1914, the Federal Government passed a law that prohibited prescrib-ing opioid drugs for recreational use. The Federal Controlled Substances Act of 1970 formulated schedules for drugs. You need to be aware of three of five schedules; I, has no current accepted medical use like heroin or marijuana, II; high abuse and dependence potential like morphine, codeine or oxycodone, and III; includes drugs with a lesser dependence and abuse liability. Hydrocodone is a schedule III drug. Valium, a relaxant is a schedule IV drug and some cough medicines are schedule V drugs. Oxycodone (Oxycotin) is a schedule II drug which means that it is potentially more habit forming than hydrocodone.

There is a difference between the descriptions of narcotic drugs and opioids. Opioids are drugs like morphine, hydrocodone etc. Narcotics are extremely addictive drugs and include heroin and other drugs that can cause sedation. Opioids act by attaching to a group of proteins called opioid receptors, found in the brain, spinal cord and gastrointestinal tract. When these drugs link to certain opioid receptors in the brain and spinal cord they can block the transmission of pain messages to the brain.

For the purposes of discussion in outlining the pharmacologic activity these compounds, the opioids will be classified as (1) agonists, (2) antagonists, and (3) mixed agonist-antagonists. All drugs bind to receptors that exist on the outer membrane of your cells.

Narcotics bind to narcotic receptors on cells in the brain and spinal cord. Opioid receptors may also be recruited on tissue cells outside of your central nervous system such as your knee following an injury. An injection of morphine into your knee may alleviate your pain.

When opioids turn on a receptor, that receptor decreases pain signals usually in your spinal cord that prevents pain signals from going to your brain. As a result, your pain perception is decreased. Experimental studies involving binding of opioids to specific receptors in the brain and spinal cord have substantiated the hypothesis that these receptors exist which mediates the actions of the opioid drugs to stop pain signals to your brain. There are two basic classes of opioid receptors called mu and kappa receptors.

Other classes exist (e.g. delta) but are not important for the discussion of your pain in this chapter. These receptors also appear to be the site of action of the endogenous (pain drugs produced by your body) opioid-like substances and have been divided into three major categories, designated mu, and kappa.

It has also been proposed that at least two subtypes of each category of opioid receptors exist. Experimental evidence suggests that activation of mu receptors (found principally at sites in the brain) is associated with analgesia, respiratory depression, euphoria, and physical dependence.

The kappa receptors (located within the spinal cord) are believed to mediate spinal analgesia, constriction of the pupil size and sedation. The other receptors may influence affective behavior, and although some physicians believe that activation of these receptors plays a role in opioid-induced analgesia. This remains controversial.

Since a number of different compounds, (e.g., certain antihistamines, some steroids, and anti-psychotics have phencyclidine) none of which are opioid in structure but can affect binding affinity for these sites. Agonistic (stimulating) opioids act as analgesics by binding to and activating both mu and kappa receptors in the brain and spinal cord.

The opioid antagonists bind to all categories of opioid receptor sites throughout the body, but fail to activate them. These compounds are not used for pain control; rather, the utility of these drugs lies in their ability to reverse an overdose of opioids including narcotics.

The compounds that comprise the mixed agonist-antagonist group are more recent additions to the clinically important opioids. These drugs are semi-synthetic derivatives of morphine, the chemical structures of which have agonistic activity at some kappa receptors but antagonistic activity at mu receptors, e.g., pentazocine, butorphanol, and nalbuphine, or partial agonistic activity at mu receptors and antagonistic activity at kappa receptors, eg. buprenorphine. All are effective analgesics since they stimulate either mu or kappa receptors.

Chemically, the opioid agonists include a number of classes of drugs, all of which have pharmacologic effects similar to those of morphine. Morphine is the oldest known drug of this class. It remains as the prototype for the opioid group and is the standard to which all other opioid analgesic drugs are compared.

Opioid drugs decrease pain but also affect all organ systems. Your pituitary gland in your brain can be adversely affected by chronic narcotic use. For example in males opioids can decrease testosterone that can cause depression and erectile dysfunction. Drowsiness and blurred vision can occur. Changes in mood can occur. An inability to concentrate can occur.

Euphoria can be experienced in 20% of individuals taking opioid drugs. Euphoria can be the cause of addiction. Opioids can stop your respiratory drive that can cause you to stop breathing. Narcotics affect your stomach by slowing down the passage of food in combination with your brain to cause nausea and vomiting. Opioids can cause a significant decrease in your blood pressure that may cause you to fall. Opioids decrease movement of the bowel resulting in constipation.

Morphine can make gall bladder disease worse by contracting a valve where the gall bladder meets the intestine called the sphincter of Oddi. Opioid drugs can result in a release of histamine from certain cell in the body that can cause itching and a rash.  As you can see opioid drugs can have side effects.

Tolerance, addiction and physical dependence can occur with opioid drugs.  Tolerance occurs when it takes more of the drug to cause the same decrease in your pain.  This is not addiction.  Patients may find that they develop tolerance to opioid pain medications and may need to have their doses increased in order to be effective. Tolerance has not been shown to lead to drug addiction.

Physical dependence is a condition that occurs when continued use of the drug is needed to prevent a withdrawal reaction.  Steady use of opioids can result in tolerance to the drugs so that higher doses must be taken to achieve the same effects. Long-term use also can lead to physical depend-ence—the body adapts to the presence of the drug and withdrawal symp-toms occur if use is reduced abruptly.

Addiction is an intense craving for an opioid and is often associated with recreational use. Signs and symptoms of addiction include yawning, sweating, restlessness, irritability, anxiety, nasal discharge, tearing, dilated pupils, gooseflesh, tremors, loss of appetite, body aches, nausea and vomit-ing, fever and chills and an increase in heart rate and blood pressure.  These symptoms last 7-10 days.

Minor symptoms can begin in 8-12 hours after the last dose of the opioid.  The more severe symptoms like nausea and vomiting begin 48-72 hours after the last dose of the drug. With respect to agonist drugs, mor-phine is the prototype.  It can be administered by mouth, rectum or by injection into muscle or vein.  It is prepared in a capsule, tablet or a liquid.

It is available by a rectal suppository as well.  This route of admin-istration is used for those patients who cannot swallow or are having severe vomiting. Hydromorphone and oxymorphone also come in the form of rectal suppositories.  The duration of action of opioids varies from drug to drug.

Sustained release morphine and oxycodone give a longer duration of action.  Immediate release drugs (eg. OXIR) give a faster onset but have a shorter duration of action.   Fentanyl, which is 75 times more potent than morphine is available in a patch and sucker, forms.

The fentanyl patch is used for severe constant pain. The pain relief is continuous. The sucker, which only comes in a raspberry flavor, is used for severe cancer pain in instances where the severe pain fluctuates. Fentora is another oral form of fentanyl.

With respect to the fentanyl pain patch, the amount of drug released is controlled by small holes in a membrane in the patch.  A larger hole permits the release of fentanyl into your body. The patches are available in different doses. The fentanyl is released for 48-72 hours. Patients with a fever can be at a risk for an overdose as the amount of fentanyl administered to your body can increase by 25% for every 30C increase in body temperature. The advantage of the patch is that patients do not have to take frequent pills during the night. The patch should be applied to a hairless surface.

Codeine is a weaker opioid that is used to treat mild pain. It may be combined with acetaminophen to make each more potent. You need to be aware that smoking tobacco can decrease the potency of Darvon and hydrocodone.

Tramadol (Ultram) is an interesting drug and may be used for moderate to moderately severe pain. It has a low abuse potential. It is not a scheduled drug. It activates mu and kappa receptors. The side effects are minimal when compared to opioid drugs. Tramadol does not produce withdrawal symptoms like opioids.

The advantage of tramadol over other drugs is that tramadol inhibits noreoinepherine and serotonin. These two substances in the brain and spinal cord also decrease pain. The opioid drugs do not have this effect. Tramadol can cause nausea dizziness and headaches. Tramadol does not lower the heart rate or blood pressure. Tramadol pro-vides pain relief similar to codeine and propoxyphene.

Buprenorphine is a semisynthetic opioid derivative of thebaine. It is a mixed partial agonist opioid receptor modulator that is used to treat opioid addiction in higher dosages, to control moderate acute pain in non-opioid-tolerant individuals in lower dosages and to control moder-ate chronic pain in even smaller doses.

Naloxone and naltrexone are drugs that reverse the respiratory effects of opioids. Naltrexone can be given orally. The only time that these drugs are given is to treat opioid intoxication. Butorphanol (Stadol) and pentazocine (Talwin) are called mixed agonist-antagonists drugs.

These drugs show receptor selectivity and these two drugs stimulate kappa recep-tors. These drugs have less opioid abuse tendencies than the agonist drugs. Opioids on the other hand work on both mu and kappa receptors. Strong opioids exist which are usually reserved for cancer patients or other patients with severe pain.

Hydromorphone (Dilaudid) and levorphanol (Levo-Droman) are eight and five times more potent than morphine. Meperidine (Demerol) is an opioid that is weaker than morphine. It is used infrequently in pain management as it can cause tremors or seizures if used on a chronic basis. Methadone is a synthetic drug similar to morphine.

The advantage of methadone for your pain management is that it does not cause euphoria. Methadone however, can cause a conduction problem in your heart. Consequently, patients have died from heart problems after being prescribed methadone. Hydrocodone and oxycodone are two opioids used for moderate to moderately severe pain. These drugs are usually combined with aspirin and acetaminophen which can potentiate the analgesic efficacy of these drugs.

Tapentadol is used to help relieve moderate to severe short-term pain (such as pain from an injury or after surgery). It also belongs to a class of drugs known as narcotic (opioid) analgesics. It works in the brain to change how your body feels and responds to pain. This medication may also be used to help relieve nerve pain (peripheral neuropathy) in people with diabetes. This medication may rarely cause abnormal drug-seeking behavior.

Another fact that you need to know is that opioid drugs can actually cause you to experience increased pain in some instances. This observation is called opioid induced pain. Many physicians are unaware of this fact. In this situation, a reduction in your dose of your medicine or stopping it can actually decrease your pain. This phenomenon can also be seen in patents that have spinal morphine drug delivery systems.

Given that no two people are alike, if you are taking any medications and begin to take nutritional supplements you should be aware that potential drug-nutrient interactions may occur and are encouraged to consult a health care professional before using any natural product. Combining certain prescription drugs and dietary supplements can lead to undesirable effects such as: diminished prescription drug effectiveness, reduced supplement effectiveness and impaired drug and/or supplement absorption.

In rats, morphine produced a significant increase in fat intake and decrease in carbohydrate intake, while naloxone led to a slight reduction in fat intake. When the two drugs were given together, a significant elevation in carbohydrate intake and reduction in fat intake were observed. Protein intake was not affected by any of the drugs. No human studies have not been done yet with respect to opioids and fat intake.[1] Another study concluded that activation of mu opioid receptors makes animals hyperphagic and selectively increases their preference for a high fat diet independent of their dietary preference.[2]

As one can see, there are many opioids that can be used for the management of your pain. The proper choice of your medication is dependent upon the magnitude of your pathology, the side effects of the drug pre-scribed, the effectiveness of the drug and your overall health.

References

1.    Marks-Kaufman R, Kanarek RB. Diet selection following a chronic morphine and naloxone regimen. Pharmacol Biochem Behav. 1990;35(3):665-669.

2.    Barnes MJ, Argyropoulos G, Bray GA. Preference for a high fat diet, but not hyperphagia following activation of mu opioid receptors is blocked in AgRP knockout mice. Brain Res. 2010;1317:100-107.

# 9. ADDICTION

Drugs are chemicals that have a profound impact on the neurochemical balance in your brain. This action affects how you feel and act. People who are suffering emotionally use drugs to escape from their problems. This can lead to drug abuse and addiction. Some physicians are afraid to prescribe scheduled drugs because of the possibility of causing addiction. Addiction is a chronic relapsing brain disease.

An addiction can occur with drugs, gambling, overeating etc. Drugs can make you euphoric. As a result, you may request more and more drugs to maintain this euphoria. Drug abuse or substance abuse, involves the repeated and excessive use of prescription or street drugs.

In one way or another, almost all drugs over stimulate the pleasure center of the brain, flooding it with the neurotransmitter dopamine which produces euphoria. That heightened sense of pleasure can be so compelling that the brain wants that feeling back, again and again.

Addiction is frequently found in people with a wide variety of mental illnesses, including anxiety disorders, unipolar and bipolar depression, schizophrenia, and borderline and other personality disorders. Methadone can be used for the treatment of pain in addicted patients.

Methadone is also an opiate that prevents users from getting high on heroin by competing with the much more potent opiates for the body's opiate receptors. Buprenophrine is another drug that is effective for the treatment of addiction and is also an analgesic.

Once your brain and body get used to the substances you are taking, you begin to require increasingly larger and more frequent doses, in order to achieve the same effect.

Narcotics such as Heroin may over-stimulate the pleasure centers of the brain producing euphoric effects that cause compulsive drug-seeking behaviors. The severities of withdrawal symptoms associated with narcotics include chills, shakes, muscle pain, nausea, vomiting, and headaches and cravings.

Drug seekers may be difficult to distinguish from true chronic pain sufferers. In general, drug seekers prefer illicit drugs such as heroin and cocaine to prescription drugs. Prescription drugs however, have advantages over illicit drugs. Third-party insurers or welfare-entitlement programs may pay for prescribed drugs. Prescription pharmaceuticals are obtained in the safety of the physician's office.

An estimated 20 percent of people in the United States have used prescription drugs for nonmedical reasons. Central nervous stimulants, depressants and opioids are prescription drugs that are frequently abused. Central nervous system depressants are used to treat anxiety, panic attacks, and sleep disorders. Examples are Nembutal (pentobarbital sodium), Valium (diazepam), and Xanax (alprazolam). Long-term use can lead to physical dependence and addiction.

Central nervous system stimulants are used to treat narcolepsy and the attention deficit/hyperactivity disorder. Examples include Ritalin (methylphenidate) and Dexedrine (dextroamphetamine). Opioids, also known as narcotic analgesics are used to treat pain. Opioids are the most commonly abused prescription drugs. Examples include morphine, codeine, OxyContin (oxycodone), Vicodin (hydrocodone) and Demerol (meperidine).

One may obtain drugs by the following means: prescription forgery, by telephone (faking to be a physician's office), multiple doctors, and indiscriminate prescribing by physicians. Pain clinicians who prescribe chronic opioids are aware that there is an illicit market for opioid analgesics. For example Oxycontin can be sold for $1.00 per milligram.

One 80 mg pill can be sold on the street for $80.00. Telephone scams occur when the drug seeker claims to be a patient of one of the other physicians in the on-call group, and asks for a prescription for an analgesic to last until they can see their regular physician. Sometimes, the drug seeker uses a telephone to impersonate a practicing physician.

Prescription forgery is a common activity among drug seekers. Drug seekers can modify a legitimate prescription to increase the dosage or quantity of an opioid. The easiest method is to increase the number of tablets on the prescription.

Multiple episodes of noncompliance raise an alert of drug seeking behavior as well as multiple episodes of prescription loss. The patient with chemical dependency loses control over drug taking. The patient cannot take medications as prescribed. The patient repeatedly reports lost or stolen medications.

The physician will notice that the drug seeker frequently requests early renewals of prescriptions. A pain physician must however, be aware that aggressive complaining about the need for more drugs may indicate inadequate pain management as opposed to drug seek-ing behavior. A patient should not be allowed to suffer. It should be understood that substance abusers can suffer from chronic pain which should be treated in a humane manner.

Unapproved use of opioids to treat another symptom such as sleep deprivation should not be tolerated.  However, the pain management physician must objectively identify a patient's pain complaint with the appropriate medical test before prescribing an opioid.  Opioid analgesics are powerful tools in the armamentarium of the pain clinician

A pain medicine physician must therefore, use safe prescribing strategies.  A physician has no legal obligation to prescribe opioid analgesics on demand.  A reasonable precaution to be taken by the pain medicine physician with an unfamiliar patient is to establish a policy of not prescribing opioid analgesics pending a complete assessment including corroboration of the patient's history.

The American Academy of Pain Medicine, the American Pain Society, and the American Society of Addiction Medicine recognize the following definitions and recommend their use.

I. Addiction

Addiction is a primary, chronic, neurobiologic disease, with genetic, psychosocial, and environmental factors influencing its development and manifestations.  It is characterized by behaviors that include one or more of the following: impaired control over drug use, compulsive use, continued use despite harm, and craving. An entity termed pseudo-addiction exists which is not true addiction.

Pseudo-addiction occurs when pain is under treated.  Pseudoaddiction resolves when the pain resolves.  Addictive behavior on the other hand, persists in spite of increasing the patient's pain medication.

II. Physical Dependence

Physical dependence is a state of adaptation that is manifested by a drug class specific withdrawal syndrome that can be produced by abrupt cessation, rapid dose reduction, decreasing blood level of the drug, and/or administration of an antagonist.

III.Tolerance

Tolerance is a state of adaptation in which exposure to a drug induces changes that result in a   diminution of one or more of the drug's effects over time. Most specialists in pain medicine and addiction medicine agree that patients treated with prolonged opioid therapy usually do develop physical dependence and sometimes develop tolerance, but do not usually develop addictive disorders.

Addiction is a primary chronic disease and exposure to opioid medications is only one of the etiologic factors in its development. Therefore, good clinical judgment must be used in determining whether the pattern of behaviors signals the presence of addiction or reflects a different issue.

Given that no two people are alike, if you are taking any medications and begin to take nutritional supplements you should be aware that potential drug-nutrient interactions may occur and are encouraged to consult a health care professional before using any natural product.

Combining certain prescription drugs and dietary supplements can lead to undesirable effects such as: diminished prescription drug effectiveness, reduced supplement effectiveness and impaired drug and/or supplement absorption.

Opioids are important in reward processes leading to addictive behavior such as self-administration of opioids and other drugs of abuse including nicotine and alcohol. Opioids are also involved in a broadly distributed neural network that regulates eating behavior, affecting both homeostatic and hedonic mechanisms.

In this sense, opioids are particularly implicated in the modulation of highly palatable foods, and opioid antagonists attenuate both addictive drug taking and appetite for palatable food. Thus, craving for palatable food could be considered as a form of opioid-related addiction.[1]

Contributing to the obesity epidemic with respect to nutrition, there is increasing evidence that overconsumption of high-fat foods may be analogous to drug addiction in that the palatability of these foods is associated with activation of specific reward pathways in the brain.[2]

References

1.          Nogueiras R, Romero-Pico A, Vazquez MJ, Novelle MG, Lopez M, Dieguez C. The opioid system and food intake: homeostatic and hedonic mechanisms. Obes Facts. 2012;5(2):196-207.

2.          Schwindinger WF, Borrell BM, Waldman LC, Robishaw JD. Mice lacking the G protein gamma3-subunit show resistance to opioids and diet induced obesity. Am J Physiol Regul Integr Comp Physiol. 2009;297(5):R1494-1502.

Pain is the most common symptom encountered in the hospitalized patient. Acute pain management is necessary following surgery, in burn patients and in sickle cell disease. Acute pain is mentioned in this book because the manner in which acute pain is treated can affect chronic pain occurrence and its management. Acute pain is the pain experienced after tissue injury from surgery, cancer or trauma.

Chronic pain is pain that continues after tissue has healed. Pain that is under treated in the hospital can lead to an increase in your blood pressure and heart rate.

Under treated acute pain may make the management of chronic pain difficult, as you may be skeptical of pain care from other physicians. You may as a result of improperly acute pain management exaggerate your symptoms to insure that you receive an adequate dose of pain medications.

Effective pain management is fundamental to quality care, and good pain control speeds recovery following surgery. Advantages of good acute pain management can be shown by increases in patient mobility and cough suppression.

Effective relief can be achieved with oral non-opioids and non-steroidal anti-inflammatory drugs. These drugs are appropriate for many post-surgical and post-traumatic pains, especially when you go home on the day of the operation.

There is an old adage that if patients can swallow it is best to take drugs by mouth. There is no evidence that non-steroidal anti-inflammatory drugs given rectally or by injection perform better than the same drug at the same dose given by mouth.. These other routes become appropriate when patients cannot swallow. Topical non-steroidal anti-inflammatory drugs are effective in acute musculoskeletal injuries.

A patient's perception of pain varies among individuals. A person's first experience with severe pain may be after surgery. At one time post-surgical pain was managed with shots of narcotic into your muscle. Postoperative pain management is now more advanced.

The goal of acute pain management is to keep a patient comfortable while avoiding opioid addiction. Inadequately treated acute pain may result in patient depression and/or anxiety. Depression can decrease your pain tolerance. This means that mild pain may be perceived as severe pain by the depressed patient. There is an ethical and humanitarian need to treat patients suffering with acute pain.

Barriers to effective pain management involve prejudice on the part of the physicians and/or patients. Patients and some physicians are afraid of opioid addiction. Addiction usually does not occur when an opioid is used short term. When considering the use of opioids for acute pain, the treating physician must consider the risks and benefits of opioid administration. The physician must however, consider the ethical responsibility of relieving a patient's pain and suffering. For severe acute pain opioids are the first line treatment.

Intermittent opioid injections can provide effective relief of acute pain. Unfortunately, adequate doses are withheld because of traditions, misconceptions, ignorance and fear. Doctors and nurses fear addiction and respiratory depression.

Addiction is not a problem with opioid use in acute pain. Irrespective of the route, opioids used for people who are not in pain, or in doses larger than necessary to control the pain, can slow or stop breathing. The key principle is to titrate the dose against the desired effect.

There is no evidence that demonstrates that one opioid is better than another. Morphine is commonly used for the treatment of acute pain. Morphine has an active metabolite, morphine-6-glucuronide.

Morphine also has a metabolite; morphine-3-glucuronide that does not provide pain relief in renal dysfunction morphine-6-glucuronide can accumulate in your body and result in a greater effect from a given dose, because it is more active than morphine. Less morphine will be needed to control your pain.

Accumulation of morphine can be a problem with unconscious intensive care patients on fixed dose schedules when renal function is compromised. Opioid adverse effects include nausea and vomiting, constipation, sedation, pruritus (itching), urinary retention and respiratory depression. There is no good evidence that the incidences of these side effects are different with different opioids.

Patient controlled analgesia is a method of pain relief that allows you to self-administer small amounts of narcotics on demand into your vein. The patient presses a button and receives a pre-set dose of opioid, from a syringe driver connected to an intravenous or subcutaneous cannula. This device delivers opioid to the same opioid receptors as an intermittent injection, but allows you to prevent delays for pain treatment.

There is little difference in outcome between efficient intermittent injections. You can select how much medication is necessary to control your pain. This method of pain relief avoids delays in your pain management. You have control over your pain.

This method of pain relief is safe because the drug delivery machine only allows you to get a specific amount of drug each hour. When it is time to discontinue your medicine, you will be given a pill. You will still have access to your drug delivery machine.

Epidural analgesia is another method for managing your pain after surgery. A small tube is placed in your back. A pump is connected to this tube to give you medicine when you need it. This pump can be programmed to give you medication like the patient controlled drug delivery system. Narcotics, local anesthetics and muscle relaxants can be placed into your body by this method.

Narcotics can also be placed into your spinal fluid. This is called intrathecal therapy and is used for acute cancer pain management. If you are having surgery on your arm or leg, s small tube can be placed in your extremity that will give a continual dose of local anesthetic.

For example if you are having surgery on your leg, a tube can be placed at the nerve that causes your pain to numb it. You can then have physical therapy without any pain. Other routes of opioid administration include intra-articular, nasal, active transdermal and inhalational administration.

Pre-emptive analgesia is used when patients have established pain prior to surgery. For example, if you have severe chronic hand and wrist pain prior to scheduled surgery, your anesthesiologist may do a nerve block to stop your pain prior to hand surgery.

The advantage of regional analgesia with a local anesthetic is that it can deliver complete pain relief by interrupting pain transmission from a specific area, so avoiding generalized drug adverse effects. This advantage is more obvious when it is possible to give further doses via a catheter, extending the duration of analgesia.

Be aware that established pain is harder to control than new pain. When chronic pain occurs, changes occur in your brain and spinal cord. These changes enhance pain perception after surgery.

Placement of a hollow tube (epidural catheter) with the administration of a local anesthetic (numbing medication) can significantly decrease your postoperative pain and may decrease your chance of developing chronic pain. Epidural infusion via a catheter can offer continuous relief after trauma or surgery, for your lower limb, spine, abdominal or chest.

The risks of associated with an epidural injection include a spinal headache, infection, hematoma or nerve damage. Some epidural infusions contain local anesthetics. Side effects of local anesthetics include a decrease in your blood pressure, motor block of your muscles, seizures, and heart rhythm disturbances. If opioids are used, side effects can include nausea and vomiting, sedation, urinary retention, respiratory depression and generalized itching.

There other types of acute pain besides post-surgical pain. Burn pain can be a result of medical treatments like dressing changes or from the thermal destruction of the tissue itself. The dead tissue must be frequently removed. This procedure is painful. Narcotics and anesthesia drugs like ketamine are necessary to control the pain.

Sickle cell disease pain can be profound as well. Acute bone destruction associated with this disease can be extremely painful and may require the administration of strong narcotics. Common sites of pain include the back, joints chest and abdomen. Narcotics may be given by mouth, but most patients require intravenous narcotics.

Given that no two people are alike, if you are taking any medications and begin to take nutritional supplements you should be aware that potential drug-nutrient interactions may occur and are encouraged to consult a health care professional before using any natural product.

Combining certain prescription drugs and dietary supplements can lead to undesirable effects such as: diminished prescription drug effectiveness, reduced supplement effectiveness and impaired drug and/or supplement absorption.

Probiotic treatment has been shown to improve bone formation, increase bone mass density and prevent bone loss. In elderly patients with a fracture of the distal radius, administration of the probiotic could greatly accelerating the healing process.[1]

Kaempferol is the most abundant polyphenol in tea, fruits, vegetables, and beans. Kaempferol was shown to attenuate the expansion of inflammatory lesions seen in gastritis and acute pancreatitis.[2] It has been reported s that a person's hydration status may also be an important factor in their perception of acute pain.[3]

References

1.      Lei M, Hua LM, Wang DW. The effect of probiotic treatment on elderly patients with distal radius fracture: a prospective double-blind, placebo-controlled randomised clinical trial. Benef Microbes. 2016:1-8.

2.      Kim SH, Park JG, Sung GH, et al. Kaempferol, a dietary flavonoid, ameliorates acute inflammatory and nociceptive symptoms in gastritis, pancreatitis, and abdominal pain. Mol Nutr Food Res. 2015;59(7):1400-1405.

3.      Bear T, Philipp M, Hill S, Mundel T. A preliminary study on how hypohydration affects pain perception. Psychophysiology. 2016;53(5):605-610.

# 11. ANTIINFLAMMATORY MEDICATIONS

Steroids are drugs used to reduce inflammatory pain such as arthritic joint pain. However, steroids may have significant side effects associated with their use. For example, steroids can cause weight gain, osteoporosis, avascular necrosis of your hips etc. Nonsteroidal anti-inflammatory drugs are commonly used to treat painful conditions. This may include a sprain strain injury, a headache, a toothache etc. Many individuals believe that these drugs are safe because many of them are sold over the counter. However, these drugs may have serious side effects in some individuals.

Hazardous molecules known as free radicals damage cells and accelerate the aging process. Free radicals are found in all hazardous chemicals including cigarette smoke. Free radicals also stimulate inflammation. The natural antidotes for free radicals are antioxidants, which include vitamins E and C and many other nutrients, particularly the many flavonoids found in vegetables, fruits, and herbs. Many antioxidants directly counteract the pro-inflammatory effects of free radicals.

Nonsteroidal anti-inflammatory drugs inhibit prostaglandins. Prostaglandins are a related family of chemicals that are produced by the cells of your body and have several important functions. They promote inflammation, pain, and cause fevers.

They are involved with the function of platelets that are necessary for the clotting of your blood, and protect the lining of your stomach from the damaging effects of acid. Prostaglandins are produced within your body's cells by the enzyme cyclooxygenase (COX). There are two of these enzymes, Cox 1 and Cox 2. However, only Cox-1 produces prostaglandins that support platelets and protect the stomach.

Nonsteroidal anti-inflammatory drugs (NSAIDs) block the Cox enzymes and reduce prostaglandins throughout your body. As a consequence, ongoing inflammation, pain, and fever are reduced. Since the prostaglandins that protect the stomach and support the platelets and blood clotting also are reduced, NSAIDs can cause ulcers in your stomach and cause bleeding. NSAIDs differ in how strongly they inhibit Cox-1 and, therefore, in their tendency to cause ulcers and promote bleeding.

Another important difference between the two enzymes is their ability to cause ulcers and bleeding. The more an NSAID blocks Cox-1, the greater is its tendency to cause ulcers and bleeding. One NSAID called Celebrex, blocks Cox-2, but has little effect on Cox-1. This drug is referred to as one of the selective Cox-2 inhibitors and therefore causes less bleeding and fewer ulcers than other NSAIDs. Aspirin is the only NSAID that is able to inhibit the clotting of blood for a prolonged period (4 to 7 days). This prolonged effect of aspirin makes it an ideal drug for preventing the blood clots that cause heart attacks and strokes.

COX-2 inhibitors do not cause your blood to not clot. This is one reason why COX-2 inhibitors are implicated in heart attacks. You should be aware that the FDA issued a public health advisory concerning use of non-steroidal anti-inflammatory drug products including those known as COX-2 selective agents.

The COX-2 selective agents like Celebrex may be associated with an increased risk of serious cardiovascular events especially when they are used for long periods of time or in very high-risk settings. The drugs Vioxx and Bextra have been taken off the market. Preliminary results from a long-term clinical trial suggest that long-term use of a non-selective NSAID; naproxen may be associated with an increased cardiovascular risk compared to placebo.

The FDA (Federal Drug Administration) stated that patients who are at a high risk of gastrointestinal bleeding, have a history of intolerance to non-selective NSAIDs, or are not doing well on non-selective NSAIDs may be appropriate candidates for COX-2 selective agents.

Non-selective NSAIDs are widely used in both over-the-counter and prescription settings. As prescription drugs, many are approved for short-term use in the treat-ment of pain and menstrual discomfort, and for longer-term use to treat the signs and symptoms of osteoarthritis and rheumatoid arthritis.

NSAIDS are classified as non-opioid analgesic drugs and are aspirin like drugs. Although the pharmacologic and toxicologic properties of these compounds are similar and all possess analgesic activity, only certain drugs are indicated specifically for the relief of pain (eg. Feldene, Voltaren, Advil, Naprosyn, Celebrex etc,). NSAIDS stop the production of prostaglandin production.

Since prostaglandins are formed and released in response to cell membrane injury, these substances have become associated with pain reactions that accompany tissue injury and inflammation. Prostaglandins sensitize pain receptors (mostly C fibers) by lowering the threshold to thermal, mechanical and chemical stimuli.

Thus, the increased pain sensations induced by prostaglandins is a localized event that allows the mediators of pain such as bradykinin, hista-mine and substance p, to exert a greater effect on pain receptors. The receptors are stimulated to a greater extent causing more pain. All of the

NSAIDS analgesics prevent the biosynthesis and release of prostaglandins by inhibition of prostaglandin cyclooxygenase, a cell membrane enzyme that is present in almost all cells. Therefore, the NSAIDS reduce the formation of prostaglandins and decrease the pain sensitivity caused by these substances. NSAIDS have analgesic, fever reducing, and anti-inflammatory effects.

Not all of the drugs are equally active, nor are all clinically useful, with respect to these effects. Dolobid (diflunisal) for example, is used exclusively as an analgesic but does not decrease a fever. With the exception of acetaminophen, aspirin, and ibuprofen, none of the other compounds are used to reduce fever.

NSAIDS are used in the treatment of various arthritic conditions such as rheumatoid arthritis, ankylosing spondylitis, osteoarthritis and acute gouty arthritis. As the particular inflammatory condition being treated is alleviated, the pain associated with the disease is also decreased. Pain associated with inflammatory diseases is effectively reduced by all of these NSAID drugs. Aspirin is the oldest NSAID.

Toradol (ketolorac) has minimal anti-inflammatory effects but has significant pain relieving effects. This observation suggests that anti-inflammatory effects are not related to pain relieving effects. NSAIDS have a ceiling affect. This means that when you take a certain dose of an NSAID, more of the NSAID will not give you more pain relief. This affect is opposite to that of opioid analgesics. They have no ceiling effects. This means that more of an opioid will increase your pain relief.

The Bayer Company in Germany discovered aspirin in the late 1800's. Aspirin is the prototype to which other NSAIDS are com-pared. The side effects of the NSAIDS should be briefly discussed. Serious side effects are rare. The liver and kidneys can be affected by high doses of NSAIDS prescribed over a long duration. Patients with forms of arthritis will require NSAIDS long term for the anti-inflammatory properties of the NSAIDS.

Gastrointestinal toxicity can occur with all NSAIDS that can lead to bleeding from the stomach and may lead to hospitalization and sur-gery as well as blood transfusions. Localized irritation of the stomach lining consti-tutes the most common adverse reaction associated NSAIDS.

Although epigastric distress is common at the lower doses, gastric and/or intestinal ulceration and bleeding will occur in only a small percent-age of patients. At higher doses of aspirin, erosive gastritis and gastrointesti-nal hemorrhage is observed more often. These effects are the result of the inhibition of cyclo-oxygenase 1 (COX-1).

You need cyclo-oxygenase 1 to form protective prostaglandins that reduce acid secretion by your stomach and promote the secretion of protective intestinal mucus.   Aspirin and other compounds with high anti-inflammatory activity, such as indomethacin, tend to elicit the highest incidence of gastrointestinal reactions.   Other NSAIDS like naproxen are considered to produce fewer and less intense gastrointestinal reactions than aspirin.

Acetaminophen is essentially devoid of these effects. Acetaminophen has some anti-inflammatory affects.   Newer NSAIDS that are specific for cyclo oxygenase 2 enzymes are safer than the rest of the NSAIDS that inhibit both cyclooxygenase 1 and 2.   Celebrex is safer on your stomach. With respect to the heart and lungs all of the NSAIDS can cause swelling in your extremities as well as increase your blood pressure.

It should be noted that all NSAIDS including ibuprofen and naproxen could be linked to an increased risk of a heart attack.   Because of this research, it is advisable to use the lowest effective dose of NSAID for the shortest time necessary, NSAIDS can cause clotting problems and make you prone to bleeding or bruising.

This is due to the inhibition of thromboxane A, formation in thrombocytes (cells in the bloodstream associated with clotting).   However, Celebrex does not cause this problem.   In other words, Celebrex is the only NSAID that does not adversely affect the blood thinning effects of aspirin.

With respect to your kidneys, sodium and water retention with extremity swelling are seen with NSAID use.   The higher the dose, the more prone you are for these side effects.   Ask your doctor about the lowest effective dose that can be prescribed for you.   If you are over sixty years of age you should be prescribed lower doses, as you may be more sensitive to NSAIDS than younger patients.

NSAIDS are excellent analgesic medications for pain in extremities, as well as for dental pain and headaches.   They are furthermore, non-addicting. NSAIDS should be used with caution in elderly patients.   If you are significantly sick (such as an intensive care patient, an NSAID can adversely affect your kidneys.   In some instances NSAIDS can cause kidney failure.

Nonsteroidal anti-inflammatory drugs (NSAIDs) are commonly used in the elderly for the treatment of fever, pain, pain associated with inflammation in rheumatoid arthritis and osteoarthritis, neuromuscular disorders, headache, and musculoskeletal conditions. Each year in the United States, people spend 5 to 10 billion dollars to purchase prescription and over-the-counter NSAIDs. Gastrointestinal side effects such as ulcers and bleeding are the most prevalent and life-threatening problems associated with NSAIDs in elderly individuals.

Specifically in the elderly, NSAIDs have become a leading cause of hospitalization in this age group and may increase the risk of death from ulceration more than four fold. NSAIDs and the new class of cyclo-oxygenase-2 selective NSAIDs continue as drugs of choice for analgesia and anti-inflammatory effects. Physiological changes of aging worsen the side-effect profile of NSAIDs in the elderly. These side effects, when added to the increased potential for drug interactions, lead to a much greater risk for adverse outcomes when NSAIDs are used in the elderly patient.

NSAIDS should be used with caution in pregnant patients as well. These drugs are not recommended during pregnancy, especially in the third trimester. While NSAIDs as a class are not direct congenital malformation drugs. They may however, cause premature closure of the fetal ductus arteriosus and also cause a reduction in maternal amniotic fluid. As a result, pregnant patients taking NSAIDS may require ultrasound monitoring by the treating obstetrician.

In addition NSAIDS may cause premature birth. Aspirin should not be used during pregnancy. Fetal bleeding could occur as a result of the inhibitory effects on the fetal platelets. Acetaminophen which does have slight anti-inflammatory properties is safe and well-tolerated during pregnancy.

The metabolic syndrome is a cluster of common pathologies: abdominal obesity linked to an excess of visceral fat, insulin resistance, dyslipidemia and hypertension. This syndrome is occurring at epidemic rates, with dramatic consequences for human health worldwide, and appears to have emerged largely from changes in our diet and reduced physical activity.

An important but not well-appreciated dietary change has been the substantial increase in fructose intake, which appears to be an important causative factor in the metabolic syndrome.

Given that no two people are alike, if you are taking any medications and begin to take nutritional supplements you should be aware that potential drug-nutrient interactions may occur and are encouraged to consult a health care professional before using any natural product.

Combining certain prescription drugs and dietary supplements can lead to undesirable effects such as: diminished prescription drug effectiveness, reduced supplement effectiveness and impaired drug and/or supplement absorption.

A high fructose intake and low magnesium diet may all be linked to the inflammatory response. Magnesium deficiency produces a clinical inflammatory syndrome characterized by leukocyte and macrophage activation, release of inflammatory cytokines, appearance of the acute phase proteins and excessive production of free radicals.

Magnesium deficiency combined with a high-fructose diet induces insulin resistance, hypertension, dyslipidemia, endothelial activation and prothrombic changes in combination with the upregulation of markers of inflammation and oxidative stress.[1]

is a broad-spectrum lipid-regulating drug used for clinical therapy of chronic high-grade inflammatory diseases.[2] The increasing prevalence of inflammatory diseases and the adverse effects associated with the long-term use of current anti-inflammatory therapies prompt the identification of alternative approaches to reestablish immune balance. Apigenin, an abundant dietary flavonoid, is emerging as a potential regulator of inflammation.[3] mango polyphenolics might be relevant as preventive agents in ulcerative colitis.[4]

Chronic inflammation in the body leads to the formation and development many diseases, e.g. atherosclerosis, diabetes, neurodegenerative diseases or cancer and others. A diet rich in flavonoid compounds and/or supplementation with these compounds not only improve the efficiency of prevention of nutrition, but also complement the medical therapy of many diseases.[5]

Intakes of fish oil and evening primrose oil may be of importance in mitigation of inflammation, disease activity, and oxidative stress biomarkers, through increased activities of antioxidant enzymes.[6]

References

1.      Yamashita T, Shoge M, Oda E, et al. The free-radical scavenger, edaravone, augments NO release from vascular cells and platelets after laser-induced, acute endothelial injury in vivo. Platelets. 2006;17(3):201-206.

2.      Montserrat-de la Paz S, Naranjo MC, Lopez S, Abia R, Muriana FJ, Bermudez B. Niacin and its metabolites as master regulators of macrophage activation. J Nutr Biochem. 2016;39:40-47.

3.      Cardenas H, Arango D, Nicholas C, et al. Dietary Apigenin Exerts Immune-Regulatory Activity in Vivo by Reducing NF-kappaB Activity, Halting Leukocyte Infiltration and Restoring Normal Metabolic Function. Int J Mol Sci. 2016;17(3):323.

4.      Kim H, Banerjee N, Barnes RC, et al. Mango polyphenolics reduce inflammation in intestinal colitis-involvement of the miR-126/PI3K/AKT/mTOR axis in vitro and in vivo. Mol Carcinog. 2016.

5.      Strzyga-Lach P, Czeczot H. [The role of flavonoids in the modulation of inflammation]. Pol Merkur Lekarski. 2016;40(236):134-140.

6.      Vasiljevic D, Veselinovic M, Jovanovic M, et al. Evaluation of the effects of different supplementation on oxidative status in patients with rheumatoid arthritis. Clin Rheumatol. 2016;35(8):1909-1915.

# 12. MUSCLE RELAXANTS

Muscle relaxants are effective for short-term symptomatic relief in patients with acute and chronic low back pain. However, the incidence of drowsiness, dizziness and other side effects is high. Muscle relaxants must be used with caution. Muscle relaxants are a useful adjunct in the treatment of patients with chronic and persistent pain. There are a number of categories in muscle relaxants, but one may broadly divide them into centrally acting muscle relaxants and peripherally acting muscle relaxants.

Central mechanisms of action include activity on the glycine receptors, as seen with the muscle relaxant properties of benzodiazepines, or on the GABA receptors, as seen with benzodiazepines and baclofen. Baclofen has been used to treat the spasticity of multiple sclerosis; it may also be used to treat muscle spasm associated with radiculopathy.

Cyclobenzaprine differs from amitriptyline by two hydrogen ions, and it retains many of the side effects of amitriptyline (e.g., dry mouth, constipation, irregular heartbeats).

Muscle relaxants are effective for short-term symptomatic relief in patients with acute and chronic low back pain. However, the incidence of drowsiness, dizziness and other side effects is high. Muscle relaxants must be used with caution.

Muscle relaxants are a useful adjunct in the treatment of patients with chronic and persistent pain. There are a number of categories in muscle relaxants, but one may broadly divide them into (1) centrally acting muscle relaxants and (2) peripherally acting muscle relaxants.

If your muscles are tense, you can have decreased oxygen in your muscle tissue that can cause you to experience pain. Muscle relaxants are drugs that decrease tension in your muscles. These drugs can be useful in pain management.

Muscle relaxants are not really a single class of drugs, but are a group of different drugs and each of these drugs can have an overall sedative effect on your body. These drugs other than dantrolene do not act directly on your muscles, but they act in your brain and are more of a total body relaxant.

Skeletal muscle relaxants are drugs that relax striated muscles (those that control your skeleton). Skeletal muscle relaxants may be used for relief of spasticity in neuromuscular diseases, such as multiple sclerosis, as well as for spinal cord injury and stroke. They may also be used for pain relief in minor strain injuries and control of the muscle symptoms of tetanus.

The muscle relaxants may be divided into only two groups, centrally acting and peripherally acting. The centrally acting group, which appears to act on the central nervous system, while only dantrolene has a direct action at the level of the nerve-muscle connection.

Dantrolene (Dantrium) has been used to prevent or treat malignant hyperthermia (severe elevation of your body temperature and muscle contractions during anesthesia) in surgery. When your muscles are tense, blood flow in your muscles can decrease. The decreased blood flow decreases your muscle oxygen level that can cause you to experience pain just as if your heart muscle has decreased oxygen following a heart attack. Decreased oxygen to your heart muscle is the reason you experience angina.

Strains, sprains, and other muscle and joint injuries can result in pain, stiffness, and muscle spasms. Muscle relaxants do not heal the injuries, but they do relax muscles and help ease discomfort. Muscle relaxants exert their effects by acting on the central nervous system. In the United States, they are available only with a physician's prescription. Several examples include; carisoprodol (Soma), cyclobenzaprine (Flexeril), and methocarbamol (Robaxin).

Most drugs come only in pill form. However, methocarbamol (Robax-in) is available in both tablet and injectable forms. Muscle relaxants are usually prescribed along with rest, exercise, physical therapy, or other treatments. One muscle relaxant, Zanaflex (tizanidine) does provide pain relief by decreasing Substance P which is one of your body's pain signal transmitters. This medication is helpful in decreasing pain associated with fibromyalgia. Although the muscle relaxant drugs may provide you with pain relief, they should never be considered a substitute for other forms of treatment like physical therapy.

Because muscle relaxants exert their effects on your central nervous system, they may potentate the effects of alcohol and other drugs. They may also add to the effects of anesthetics, including those used for dental procedures. For this reason, anyone who takes these drugs should not drive; operate machinery, or any activity that might be dangerous.

People with certain medical conditions or who are taking certain other medicines can have problems if they take muscle relaxants. Diabetics should be aware that metaxalone (Skelaxin) may cause false test results on one type of test that detects sugar in your urine. Patients with epilepsy should be cautioned that taking the muscle relaxant methocarbamol might increase the likelihood of seizures.

Common side effects of muscle relaxants are visual changes, such as double vision or blurred vision; dizziness; lightheadedness; drowsiness; and dry mouth. These problems usually go away as your body adjusts to the drug and do not require medical treatment. Methocarbamol and chlorzoxazone may cause temporary color changes in your urine.  Other side effects are stomach cramps, nausea and vomiting, constipation, diarrhea, hiccups, clumsiness or unsteadiness, confusion, nervousness, restlessness, irritability, flushed or red face, headache, heartburn, weakness, trembling, and sleep problems.

More serious side effects are not common, but may occur. Anyone who experiences breathing problems, facial swelling, fainting, unusually fast or unusually slow heartbeat, fever, tightness in the chest, rash, itching, hives, burning, stinging, red, or bloodshot eyes, or unusual thoughts or dreams after taking muscle relaxants should seek medical help promptly.

Parafon Forte can cause liver pathology (injury) in some individuals. The reaction is rare, but you can develop the following symptoms: fever, rash, loss of appetite, nausea, vomiting, fatigue, pain in the upper right part of the abdomen, dark urine, or yellow skin or eyes.

Muscle relaxants may interact with some other medicines. The effects of a drug may either be lessened or potentiated.  When this occurs, the effects of one or both of the drugs may change or the risk of side effects may be greater with either drug.

Anyone taking muscle relaxants should let their physician know all other medicines, including over-the-counter or nonprescription medicines that he or she is taking. Some patients for example,receive muscle relaxants from an emergency department.  They may not tell their treating physician. If they develop side effects, the primary care physician would not know what is causing any new symptoms.

Most muscle relaxants are centrally acting.  Central mechanisms of action include activity on the glycine receptors, as seen with the muscle relaxant properties of benzodiazepines, or on the GABA receptors, as seen with benzodiazepines and baclofen. Baclofen has been used to treat the spasticity of multiple sclerosis; it may also be used to treat muscle spasm associated with radiculopathy. This indication is not approved by the Food and Drug Administration (FDA) because the primary activity for this drug has been for myelopathies.

Metaxalone has a role, as do other muscle relaxants, such as carisoprodol and methocarbamol. Cyclobenzaprine (Flexeril) has atropine-like side effects. Cyclobenzaprine differs from amitriptyline by two hydrogen ions, and it retains many of the side effects of amitriptyline (e.g., dry mouth, constipation, irregular heartbeats

Some of these muscle relaxant drugs are antispasticity medications used to treat muscle spasms and are usually associated with disorders of your nervous system. A muscle spasm is an involuntary increase in your muscle tone that that occurs when you stretch your muscle. The cause of the spasm is not known but may be related to a decrease in your body's nervous system's ability to be able to control muscle contractions. Drugs that decrease spasms are called antispasmodic drugs and include drugs like Valium (benzodiazepine), baclofen (Lioresal), Zanaflex (tizanidine) or dantrolene. Each of these drugs can exert their effects for a long time. Shorter acting medications will be described below.

Botulism toxin administered into your muscle can decrease pain from muscle spasms or muscle dysfunction. These toxins (7 total A-G) prevent release of a chemical called acetylcholine from the nerve ending that goes to your muscle. This action can stop muscle spasms. Botulism toxins A and B are commonly used in a medical practice. These toxins can be used to manage pain associated with whiplash disorders, some headaches, torticolis and low back pain. Botulism toxin can relieve your pain for 3 months.It can take two weeks for the toxin to exert its effects. Botulism toxin injections can cause you to experience mild side effects. These effects may be a fever or mild joint pain.

Benzodiazepines are used for anxiety and seizure treatment, but Valium and Klonopin can both be used for muscle relaxation. These drugs exert their effects by acting in your spinal cord. These drugs are useful if you have a history of a spinal cord injury. These drugs can last for a long time once they have been introduced into your body. Valium should not be used long term. You should know Valium is a depressant and can worsen depression associated with chronic pain.

Baclofen is another powerful drug that works in your spinal cord. This drug is frequently used in patients with spinal cord injury or multiple sclerosis. Baclofen causes less sedation than benzodiazipines. However baclofen can cause some drowsiness. A sedative is a medicine used to treat restlessness.

A pump with tubing placed into your spinal cord can administer baclofen continuously throughout your spinal fluid. Dantrolene affects the muscle spasm by direct action on the muscle itself. It is used in spinal cord injuries and for the treatment of spasms associated with cerebral palsy.

Tizanidine (Zanaflex) exerts its effects on your central nervous system. It is frequently used for the treatment of muscle spasms associated with rheumatoid arthritis. This drug also decreases substance P that is a pain neurotransmitter.

Because this drug can decrease your blood pressure, you should use it with caution if you have a history of hypertension. The drugs mentioned above can have a long duration. Other drugs are available that have shorter actions. These types of drugs are used for short periods following muscle injuries. These drugs may also be used following surgery. They are not used to treat muscle spasms.

Carisoprodol (Soma) has sedative properties as well as muscle relaxant properties. This drug should be used for muscle pain. It will not however, relieve muscle spasms. This drug furthermore, may decrease your ability to fall asleep. Methocarbamol (Robaxin) is a sedative and decreases muscle pain by its sedative action. It has no muscle relaxant effects.

Cyclobenzaprine is a drug that is chemically related in structure to amitriptyline (Elavil). This drug does not act on muscles but exerts its effects on your brain. It causes sedation. However, this drug can reduce muscle pain and tenderness. Remember that all muscle relaxant drugs may cause severe sedation. You should not drive a car or operate machinery when taking muscle relaxants.

Baclofen, when administered into your spinal fluid, may cause severe central nervous system (CNS) depression with cardiovascular collapse and respiratory failure. All of the drugs mentioned can have serious side effects. Diazepam (Valium) may be highly addictive. It is a controlled substance under federal law. Valium can be a tranquilizer (a drug that has a calming effect and is used to treat anxiety and emotional tension).

Dantrolene has a potential to cause liver damage. The incidence of hepatitis is related to the amount of drug that you have taken, but may occur even with a short period of small doses. Hepatitis has been most frequently observed between the third and twelfth months of therapy. The risk of liver injury appears to be greater in women, in patients over 35 years of age and in patients taking other medications in addition to dantrolene.

If you are taking certain muscle relaxants and experience purple colored urine, you do not have a serious illness. For example, methocarbamol and chlorzoxazone may cause harmless color changes in your urine such as orange or reddish-purple with chlorzoxazone and purple, brown, or green with methocarbamol. Your urine will return to its normal color when you stop taking the medicine. Because each of these drugs can cause sedation, they should be used with caution with other drugs including alcohol that may also cause drowsiness.

Drugs that inhibit the metabolism of Valium in your liver may increase the activity of the diazepam (Valium). These drugs include: cimetidine, oral contraceptives, disulfiram, fluoxetine, isoniazid, ketoconazole, metoprolol, propoxyphene, propranolol, and valproic acid. In females dantrolene may have an interaction with estrogens. The rate of liver damage in women over the age of 35 who were taking estrogens is higher than in other groups.

Given that no two people are alike, if you are taking any medications and begin to take nutritional supplements you should be aware that potential drug-nutrient interactions may occur and are encouraged to consult a health care professional before using any natural product. Combining certain prescription drugs and dietary supplements can lead to undesirable effects such as: diminished prescription drug effectiveness, reduced supplement effectiveness and impaired drug and/or supplement absorption.

Fibromyalgia syndrome is a common, chronic musculoskeletal disorder of unknown etiology. While available therapy is often disappointing, most patients can be helped with a combination of medication, exercise and maintenance of a regular sleep schedule. Adding nutritional supplements derived from the unicellular green alga, Chlorella pyrenoidosa, produced improvements in the clinical and functional status in patients with moderately severe symptoms of the fibromyalgia syndrome[1]

There is accumulating evidence that selenium plays an important role in human nutrition. A reported case report indicated that severe muscle pain disappeared after four weeks of selenium treatment.[2]

Short-term supplementation of Montmorency powdered tart cherries surrounding a single bout of resistance exercise, appears to be an effective dietary supplement to attenuate muscle soreness, strength decrement during recovery, and markers of muscle catabolism in resistance trained individuals.[3] These cherries reduced immune and inflammatory stress, better maintained redox balance, and increased performance in aerobically trained individuals as well.[4]

It has also been reported that consumption of black currant nectar by a complex series of mechanisms, alcohol adversely affects skeletal muscle. In addition to the mechanical changes to muscle, there are important metabolic consequences, by virtue of the fact that skeletal muscle is 40% of body mass and an important contributor to whole-body protein turnover. Prior to and after a bout of eccentric exercise attenuates muscle damage and inflammation exercise-induced muscle damage[5]

On the other hand, by a complex series of mechanisms, alcohol adversely affects skeletal muscle. In addition to the mechanical changes to muscle, there are important metabolic consequences, by virtue of the fact that skeletal muscle is 40% of body mass is an important contributor to whole-body protein turnover.[6]

Skeletal muscle disorders manifested by muscle pain, fatigue, proximal weakness, and serum creatine kinase elevation have also been reported in patients with selenium deficiency.[7]

Watermelon is rich in L-citrulline, an effective precursor of L-arginine.[7] There is a beneficial effect of watermelon pomace juice as a functional food for increasing arginine availability, reducing serum concentrations of cardiovascular risk factors, improving glycemic control, and ameliorating vascular dysfunction in obese animals with type-II diabetes.[7]

An arginine and antioxidant-containing supplement increased the anaerobic threshold at both week one and week three in elderly cyclists. This study indicated a potential role of L-arginine and antioxidant supplementation in improving exercise performance in elderly cyclists.[8] Skeletal muscle disorders manifested by muscle pain, fatigue, proximal weakness, and serum creatine kinase elevation have also been reported in patients with selenium deficiency.[9]

References

1.      Merchant RE, Carmack CA, Wise CM. Nutritional supplementation with Chlorella pyrenoidosa for patients with fibromyalgia syndrome: a pilot study. Phytother Res. 2000;14(3):167-173.

2.      Shu H. [Human selenium deficiency during total parenteral nutrition support (a case report)]. Zhongguo Yi Xue Ke Xue Yuan Xue Bao. 1989;11(1):74-76.

3.      Levers K, Dalton R, Galvan E, et al. Effects of powdered Montmorency tart cherry supplementation on an acute bout of intense lower body strength exercise in resistance trained males. J Int Soc Sports Nutr. 2015;12:41.

4.      Levers K, Dalton R, Galvan E, et al. Effects of powdered Montmorency tart cherry supplementation on acute endurance exercise performance in aerobically trained individuals. J Int Soc Sports Nutr. 2016;13:22.

5.      Hutchison AT, Flieller EB, Dillon KJ, Leverett BD. Black Currant Nectar Reduces Muscle Damage and Inflammation Following a Bout of High-Intensity Eccentric Contractions. J Diet Suppl. 2016;13(1):1-15.

6.      Preedy VR, Adachi J, Ueno Y, et al. Alcoholic skeletal muscle myopathy: definitions, features, contribution of neuropathy, impact and diagnosis. Eur J Neurol. 2001;8(6):677-687.

7.      Chariot P, Bignani O. Skeletal muscle disorders associated with selenium deficiency in humans. Muscle Nerve. 2003;27(6):662-668.

8.   Wu G, Collins JK, Perkins-Veazie P, et al. Dietary supplementation with watermelon pomace juice enhances arginine availability and ameliorates the metabolic syndrome in Zucker diabetic fatty rats. J Nutr. 2007;137(12 ):2680-2685.

9.  Chariot P, Bignani O. Skeletal muscle disorders associated with selenium deficiency in humans. Muscle Nerve. 2003;27(6):662-668.):2680-2685.

# 13. ANTICONVULSANTS

Anticonvulsant drugs have been used for the management of neuropathic (damaged nerves) pain since the 1960s. These drugs interfere with the total number of pain signals that travel to your brain. The clinical impression is that they are useful for chronic neuropathic (nerve damage) pain, especially when the pain is lancinating or burning. Pain is usually the natural consequence of tissue injury resulting in approximately forty million medical appointments per year. In general, following most injuries, as the healing process commences, the pain and tenderness associated with your injury will resolve. Unfortunately, some individuals experience pain without an obvious injury or suffer pain that persists for months or years after their initial injury. This pain condition is neuropathic in nature and accounts for a large number of patients presenting to pain clinics with chronic pain.

Following any tissue injury (nerve, muscle, bone, etc.) your nervous system sounds an alarm to your brain to make you aware that you have been injured. Rather than your nervous system functioning properly to sound an alarm regarding tissue injury, in neuropathic pain, the peripheral or central nervous systems are malfunctioning and become the cause of the pain. In other words, after your nerve has healed it may still transmit pain signals. An example is a car alarm. The alarm will sound if your vehicle is being tampered with. This is normal. Now imagine that your alarm sounds when no one is near your car. Somehow there is a short circuit. The same occurs within your nervous system.

Neuropathic pain is a complex, pain state that usually is accompanied by nerve injury. With neuropathic pain, the nerve fibers themselves may be damaged, dysfunctional or injured. These damaged nerve fibers send incorrect signals to other pain centers. The impact of nerve injury includes a change in nerve function both at the site of injury and areas around the injury. Symptoms may include: shooting and burning pain and tingling and numbness.

In order to understand the effects of antiseizure drugs, you need to be aware that these drugs can block the ion (calcium and sodium) channels that are present throughout your nervous system. Ion channels are pore-forming proteins that help to establish and control a small electrical gradient between the inside and outside of your nerve cells. When ions flow in and out of your neuron, this electrical gradient ceases and pain signals subsequently cease to be transmitted to your brain. Calcium and sodium channned anticonvulsant drugs block the pores or channels. When these drugs drop off of these channels, you will experience pain again.

Antiseizure drugs are frequently used in pain management. It is not known exactly how anticonvulsants work to reduce pain. They may block the flow of pain signals from your brain and spinal cord. Some anticonvulsant drugs may work better than others for certain conditions. Neuropathic pain, is a form of chronic pain caused by an injury to or a disease of your peripheral or central nervous system. It does not respond well to traditional pain therapies like opioids or nonsteroidal anti-inflammatory drugs.

In neuropathic pain, it has shown that a number of pathophysiological and biochemical changes take place in the nervous system as a result of an insult to a nerve. This property of the nervous system to adapt to external stimuli plays a crucial role in the onset and maintenance of pain symptoms. Carbamazepine (Tegretol), the first anticonvulsant studied in clinical trials, probably alleviates pain by decreasing conductance in sodium channels and inhibits ectopic nerve discharges. Results from clinical trials have been positive in the treatment of trigeminal neuralgia, painful diabetic neuropathy and postherpetic neuralgia with this medication.

Gabapentin (Neurontin) and pregabilin (Lyrica) have the most clearly demonstrated analgesic effects for the treatment of neuropathic pain, specifically for the treatment of painful diabetic neuropathy and postherpetic neuralgia. Based on the positive results of these studies and its favorable adverse effect profile, gabapentin or pregabilin should be considered the first choice of therapy for neuropathic pain. Evidence for the efficacy of phenytoin as an antinociceptive agent is, at best, weak to modest. Lamotrigine (Lamictal) on the other hand has good potential to modulate and control neuropathic pain.

There is a potential for phenobarbital, clonazepam, valproic acid, topiramate, pregabalin and tiagabine to have antihyperalgesic and antinociceptive activities based on result in animal models of neuropathic pain, but the efficacy of these drugs in the treatment of human neuropathic pain has not yet been fully determined in clinical trials. The role of anticonvulsant drugs in the treatment of neuropathic pain is evolving and has been clearly demonstrated with gabapentin and carbamazepine. Further advances in our understanding of the mechanisms underlying neuropathic pain syndromes and well-designed clinical trials should further the opportunities to establish the role of anticonvulsants in the treatment of neuropathic pain.

If you have had a direct injury to one of your nerves, you may benefit from an anticonvulsant drug. The clinical impression is that these drugs are useful for the treatment of chronic neuropathic pain, especially when the pain is lancinating or burning.    There are seven drugs that are useful in neuropathic (nerve injury) pain; pregabilin (Lyrica), gabapentin (Neurontin), carbamazipine (Tegretol), valproic acid (Depakote), clonazepamm (Klonopin), phenytoin (Dilantin) ,zonisamide (Zonegran)) and lamotrigine (Lamictal).

Neurontin is an effective drug for the treatment of neuropathic pain but Lyrica is becoming widely used in the management of many pain syndromes.  It has fewer side effects than other anticonvulsant drugs.  These drugs can be useful for the treatment of shingles, diabetic neuropathy and fibromyalgia. Reflex Sympathetic Dystrophy, diabetic neuropathy migraine headaches, sciatica, radiculitis, and pain associated with multiple sclerosis may respond to either of these drugs.

If you experience sharp shooting pain, these drugs may be helpful in decreasing your pain.  If you experience side effects from either drug, other anticonvulsant medications are available.    Oxcarbazepine (Trileptal), lamotrigine (Lamictal), topiramate (Topamax), and zonisamide (Zonegran) may also be effective in reducing pain caused by diabetic neuropathy and postherpetic neuralgia. Lyrica is now FDA approved in 2007 for the treatment of fibromyalgia.

Anticonvulsant drugs are effective in the treatment of chronic neuropathic pain but were not initially thought to be useful in the management of postoperative pain. However, similar to any nerve injury, surgical tissue injury is known to produce neuroplastic changes leading to spinal sensitization and the expression of nerve induced pain. Gabapentin (Neurontin) may decrease post-surgical pain. The pharmacological effects of anticonvulsant drugs, which may be important in the modulation of these postoperative neural changes, include suppression of sodium channel, calcium channel and glutamate receptor activity at peripheral, spinal and supraspinal sites.

Your doctor may obtain a complete blood count and liver tests before prescribing some of these anticonvulsant drugs (e.g. Tegretol).  Your doctor will give you a 4 to 6 week trial of the drug.  It may take the medication this length of time to exert its effects. Therefore, if you have no pain relief after several days you should not stop the drug that was prescribed to you.

Because it takes your body time to adjust to one of these medications, your doctor must adhere to the phrase "begin low and proceed slow" which means that you should be prescribed a low dose and this dose may be increased gradually over days to weeks. Anticonvulsant drugs are effective in the treatment of chronic pain but may also be useful for pain management following surgery.

Similar to any nerve injury, surgical tissue injury is known to produce changes leading to spinal cord sensitization which can cause you to have pain after surgery. Gabapentin has been shown to decrease post-surgery pain. Pregabilin is effective for the treatment of diabetic neuropathy and shingles.

Pregabilin binds to calcium channels of nerves, which results in a reduction of your pain. Some insurance plans do not pay for Lyrica because it is new and relatively expensive. However, it has been shown to be more cost effective than gabapentin. This drug can cause dizziness, blurred vision, drowsiness, weight gain and swelling of your legs. This medication may decrease your platelet count as well.

Some anticonvulsant medicines can cause a decrease in your platelets which can interfere with your ability to form a blood clot. If your platelets are too low, you will bruise easily. Gabapentin is effective for the management of oral phantom pain following a tooth extraction. Gabapentin binds to nerve calcium channels. The drug is useful in most nerve injury pain disorders. An average dose is 300 mg taken three times a day.

Tegretol is a drug that is chemically related to amitriptyline. It prevents repetitive discharges of your nerves. This medication works on sodium channels in your painful nerves. Inhibition of these sodium channels can decrease your pain sensations. An average dose is 200 mg every day. Side effects include dizziness, drowsiness, blurred vision and nausea. This medication can cause various forms of anemia and liver damage. As a result, your doctor will obtain a blood count and liver tests.

Tegretol has been shown to be effective for the treatment of trigeminal neuralgia (facial pain). Depakote is given in a dose of 250 mg twice a day. This medication can cause you to have liver failure. Your doctor will monitor your liver function closely. This medicine is used when the other anti convulsant medications have been tried but failed to provide pain relief. Side effects of this drug include nausea, vomiting loss of appetite and diarrhea. Tremors and sedation may also be associated with this medication.

Klonopin may be useful for the treatment of pain associated with the burning mouth syndrome. Klonipin is useful also for the treatment of lancinating pain associated with the phantom limb syndrome. The drug may also be useful for migraine headache prophylaxis and for the treatment of trigeminal neuralgia (facial pain). The usual dose is 1 mg per day. Side effects include mood disturbances and delirium. Lethargy and sedation may also be seen. This drug has a significant sedative effect. It should be initially only taken at bedtime.

Dilantin alters sodium, calcium and potassium channels in your nerves. An average dose is 300 mg three times a day. The number of side effects associated with this drug is significant. Liver damage can occur and the drug can decrease your folic acid level in your bloodstream. A decrease in your folic acid blood level may actually cause your nerves in your arms and legs to have burning sensations.

Zonegran's mechanisms of action suggest that it could be effective in controlling neuropathic pain symptoms. It also decreases sodium channel activity on the sodium channels of your nerves.   Side effects can include a decrease in your blood sodium levels, kidney stones, visual difficulties and secondary angle-closure glaucoma.

A typical dose of this medication is   300 mg per day. Side effects related to this drug include agitation, anxiety, ataxia, confusion, depression, difficulty concentrating, headache, difficulty sleeping, memory problems, stomach pain as well as liver pathology. This medication may also cause weight loss. A dry mouth and flu like syndrome may also be associated with this drug.

Lamictal also exerts its effects on sodium channels. This drug decreases the release of some pain-causing chemical from the ends of your nerves. The reason why you develop chronic pain after having acute nerve injury pain remains unclear. However, it is believed that Lamictal in addition to some of the other drugs mentioned may prevent this transformation. A typical dose will be 200 mg twice a day after starting at a low dose and going to 200 mg slowly. Adverse effects related to this drug include headaches, dizziness, blurred vision and nausea and vomiting. This medication may be of benefit for the treatment of pain associated with Reflex Sympathetic Dystrophy.

Given that no two people are alike, if you are taking any medications and begin to take nutritional supplements you should be aware that potential drug-nutrient interactions may occur and are encouraged to consult a health care professional before using any natural product. Combining certain prescription drugs and dietary supplements can lead to undesirable effects such as: diminished prescription drug effectiveness, reduced supplement effectiveness and impaired drug and/or supplement absorption.

There is evidence suggesting that omega-3 fatty acids may have neuroprotective and anticonvulsant effects and, accordingly, may have a potential use in the treatment of epilepsy.[1]

One might expect that omega-3 fatty acids may also be effective in decreasing the intensity of neuropathic pain.

Honey is the only insect-derived natural product with therapeutic, traditional, spiritual, nutritional, cosmetic, and industrial value. In addition to having excellent nutritional value, honey is a good source of physiologically active natural compounds. Honey may decrease pain associated with nerve inflammation. The ultimate biochemical impact of honey on specific neuro-degenerative and neuroinflammation remains to be studied.[2]

Neuropathic pain is one of the most common complications of diabetes mellitus. Curcumin can be considered as a new therapeutic potential for the treatment of diabetic neuropathic pain and the activation of opioid system may be involved in the antinociceptive effect of curcumin.[3]

Dietary therapy with antioxidants could be considered as a new effective strategy in the long term for CPP, and may be better accepted by patients.[4]

References
1.      Tejada S, Martorell M, Capo X, Tur JA, Pons A, Sureda A. Omega-3 Fatty Acids in the Management of Epilepsy. Curr Top Med Chem. 2016;16(17):1897-1905.
2.      Mijanur Rahman M, Gan SH, Khalil MI. Neurological effects of honey: current and future prospects. Evid Based Complement Alternat Med. 2014;2014:958721.
3.      Banafshe HR, Hamidi GA, Noureddini M, Mirhashemi SM, Mokhtari R, Shoferpour M. Effect of curcumin on diabetic peripheral neuropathic pain: possible involvement of opioid system. Eur J Pharmacol. 2014;723:202-206.
4.      Sesti F, Capozzolo T, Pietropolli A, Collalti M, Bollea MR, Piccione E. Dietary therapy: a new strategy for management of chronic pelvic pain. Nutr Res Rev. 2011;24(1):31-38.

Antidepressant drugs are chemicals that go to your nerve connection areas in your brain and spinal cord. Neurons are not physically connected. Signals are transmitted by chemicals that go from one nerve ending to another. These drugs are chemicals that can attenuate the total number of pain signals that go to your brain. As a result you experience less pain. Side effects such as dizziness and sedation caused by high doses of amitriptyline (Elavil) cause doctors to increase doses of antidepressants very gradually over several weeks. Initially only low doses of antidepressants like Elavil are needed. However, the dose needed to control pain may need to increase over time.

The analgesic properties of anti-depressant drugs were at one time felt to be related to the alleviation of depression, which can often accompany persistent chronic pain. However, several anti-depressants have been found to reduce pain symptoms in patients' not experiencing depression. These agents are now believed to have primary analgesic abilities, which are most likely related to their effects on certain chemicals within your body. Cymbalta is one example. The efficacy of both serotonin and norepinephrine selective anti-depressants would suggest that effects on pain pathways which involve increases of either of these transmitters might contribute to analgesia.

Other suggested mechanisms of analgesia involve the antihistamine properties of some agents, increased endorphin secretion, and an increased density of cortical calcium channels. Antidepressant drugs can increase two chemicals in your brain and spinal cord that can decrease the number of pain signals that go to these structures. These chemicals are called serotonin and norepinepherine that were previously mentioned in this paragraph.

A tricyclic antidepressant drug used commonly for pain is amitriptyline (Elavil). This agent can cause constipatin and dry mouth, and some patients complain of dizziness when they stand quickly (orthos-tatic hypotension). Sedation and tremors may also occur. Weight gain and sexual dysfunction have been also been reported. Some people even complain of a craving for chocolate. An overdose of tricyclic antidepressants or related drugs may cause you to experience a dangerous and even fatal abnormality of your heart rhythm.

Elavil taken in combination with opioids can cause more constipation than either of the drugs used alone. No antidepressant drug should be stopped abruptly without the advice of a doctor. When stopped suddenly, anxiety, vivid dreams, nausea, vomiting, and dizziness may result. Because of the frequent side effects associated with tricyclic antidepressants. A newer class of antidepressant drugs called selective serotonin reuptake inhibitors (SSRIs) with fewer side effects is starting to take the place of Elavil. You do need to know however, that Elavil may have an effect on acid production in your stomach. Some of these drugs can actually decrease acid production and be of some benefit in patients who suffer from ulcers, reflux, or gastritis.

An antidepressant that is effective for some forms of pain is a combination serotonin and norepinepherine inhibitor called Cymbalta (duloxetine). This drug is effective in decreasing pain associated with diabetes called diabetic neuropathy. Cymbalta however, can make you sleepy and impair your thinking in some situations.

Another class of antidepressants is monoamine oxidase inhibitors (MAOIs). This class of antidepressant drugs is used for significant depression and is not usually used for pain management. MAOI'S drugs have a high incidence of side effects and overdoses can be lethal. These drugs increase the appetite of some patients. This class of drug increases the concentration of epinephrine, norepinephrine, and dopamine in your central nervous system, and when combined with foods such as cheese and wine high in tyramine may cause severe hypertension. For this reason, MAOIs should not be used by people with preexisting hypertension.

Side effects of MAOIs include constipation, nausea, vomiting, dry mouth, drowsiness, and dizziness. Sexual dysfunction may occur. If a MAOI is taken with meperidine (Demerol), a significant and potential-ly lethal elevation in body temperature can occur. MAOIs can also be associated with liver damage. Blood tests that assess liver function should be monitored routinely when anyone is taking any of these medications. Examples of MAOIs include Marplan and Parnate. The only time that a pain-management doctor usually sees a patient taking these drugs is when another doctor who was treating the patient for severe depression refers a patient.

You should be aware of some of the drugs in the selective serotonin reuptake inhibitors (SSRIs) class. The first drug of this class was fluoxetine (Prozac), introduced in 1987. Overall, this class of drugs causes fewer side effects than the tricyclic antidepressants or the MAOIs. The SSRIs exert their pain modulating and antidepressant effect by increasing serotonin levels in the central nervous system. This neurochemical is extremely valuable in reducing pain. Other SSRIs include piroxitine (Paxil), sertraline (Zoloft), and fluvoxamine (Luvox).

A SSRI, venlafaxine (Effexor), has been studied for its pain-modulating effects in chronic pain situations. This medication been shown to be effective in the control of pain in many painful disorders. The selective serotonin reuptake inhibitor class of drugs can cause nausea and diarrhea. Jitteriness and lack of sleep have also been reported as side effects in a small number of patients. Other individuals complain of sedation after taking this medication. If sedation is a problem, the medication should be taken only in the evening. The drug can be used as a nonaddicting sleep aid. A decreased libido is occasionally associated with this class of drugs.

Some reports exist that Prozac may lead a depressed patient to commit suicide. The drug itself does not cause suicide tendencies. Severely depressed patients can frequently have strong suicidal ideations and probably should be hospitalized while antidepressant medications were started. An individual who is sincere about committing suicide should be placed immediately under the care of a psychiatrist.

Be aware that SSRIs can decrease the efficacy of the opioid analgesics hydrocodone or oxycodone if taken in combinations with these agents. Both opioids are broken down in the liver to morphine, a chemical reaction that can be slowed by the SSRIs. As a result, less morphine is produced for pain relief.

A selective serotonin reuptake inhibitor, escitalopram oxlate (Lexapro), is now available to patients that do not affect liver metabolism. This medication does not interfere with the transformation of oxycodone and hydrocodone to morphine. Consequently, its use with these drugs will not decrease the efficacy of the opioid prescribed. Patients must be told that the selective serotonin reuptake inhibitors can cause generalized muscle pain in a small number of patients. Muscle pain is not associated with tricyclic antidepressant use.

Trazodone (Desyrel) is essentially in its own antidepressant class and is known as an "atypical antidepressant" medicine. Like the other classes of antidepressants, this drug exerts its effect by increasing serotonin in your brain and spinal cord. It is not as potent as the tricyclic antidepressants but it does cause drowsiness and may be used to enhance sleep. Side effects include dizziness and dry mouth. Priapism, a painful, persistent erection, is one of the most serious side effects of this drug in males and may precipitate a visit to an emergency room for treatment.

Studies have demonstrated that antidepressants can lessen the pain of the following syndromes in many patients: phantom pain, acute herpes zoster, post-herpetic neuralgia, cancer pain, cluster headaches, migraine headaches, reflex sympathetic dystrophy, and tension-type headaches. Is one class of antidepressant more effective than another? The drug of choice depends on the incidence of side effects as well as the effectiveness of the drug.

The occurrence of serious adverse effects resulting from antidepressant administration is low. While cardiac side effects are uncommon, tricyclic antidepressants are contraindicated in those individuals with heart failure or serious cardiac conduction abnormalities. Orthostatic hypotension (decrease in blood pressure following standing) is the most frequent cardiovascular adverse effect, and the elderly are particularly at risk. Nortriptyline and desipramine have been found to induce fewer side effects and are less sedating.

While antidepressant drugs have been demonstrated as useful adjuncts in the treatment of pain, their analgesic mechanism remains unclear. Initial dosing should be low and then slowly increased to minimize side effects. When taken at night, the sedating properties of these agents can be beneficial in those pain patients experiencing difficulty with sleep.

Nutrition is one of the most important modifiable determinants for and consequences of both mental and physical heath. Depression has become an increasingly important public health issue.

Given that no two people are alike, if you are taking any medications and begin to take nutritional supplements you should be aware that potential drug-nutrient interactions may occur and are encouraged to consult a health care professional before using any natural product. Combining certain prescription drugs and dietary supplements can lead to undesirable effects such as: diminished prescription drug effectiveness, reduced supplement effectiveness and impaired drug and/or supplement absorption.

The question on whether undernutrition remains linked to depressive symptoms, considering the effect of deficiencies of vitamin B12 and folate, is of practical relevance because they are potentially preventable and treatable. In a previous study, a decrease in folate but not vitamin B12 contributed to depression.[1]

It has been shown that in major mental illnesses such as schizophrenia, depression and Alzheimer's disease, nutritional deficiencies at cellular level are implicated.[2] Nutritional components that may be beneficial for mental health are omega-3 fatty acids, phospholipids, cholesterol, niacin, folate, vitamin B6, and vitamin B12. Saturated fat and simple sugar are considered detrimental to cognitive function.

Evidence on the effect of cholesterol is conflicting; however, in general, blood cholesterol levels are negatively associated with the risk of depression.[3]

There is evidence of decreased depression risk among women with higher intakes of vitamin B6 from food, which was dependent on total energy intake, and among men with higher intakes of B12 from food, independently of energy intake.[4]

The regulation of the calcium serum level seems to be affected in the luteal phase of the menstrual cycle and the sodium and magnesium ions influence some psychological pathology (anxiety and depression) in females. [5] Folic acid depletion furthermore lay may be associated with depression.[6]

References

1.      Brito Noronha M, Almeida Cunha N, Agra Araujo D, Flaminio Abrunhosa S, Nunes Rocha A, Freitas Amaral T. Undernutrition, Serum Vitamin B12, Folic Acid and Depressive Symptoms in Older Adults. Nutr Hosp. 2015;32(1):354-361.

2.      Zamora Navarro S, Perez Llamas F. [Importance of sucrose in cognitive functions: knowledge and behavior]. Nutr Hosp. 2013;28 Suppl 4:106-111.

3.      Lim SY, Kim EJ, Kim A, Lee HJ, Choi HJ, Yang SJ. Nutritional Factors Affecting Mental Health. Clin Nutr Res. 2016;5(3):143-152.

4.      Gougeon L, Payette H, Morais JA, Gaudreau P, Shatenstein B, Gray-Donald K. Intakes of folate, vitamin B6 and B12 and risk of depression in community-dwelling older adults: the Quebec Longitudinal Study on Nutrition and Aging. Eur J Clin Nutr. 2016;70(3):380-385.

5.      dos Santos LA, de Azeredo VB, Eloy Chaves Barbosa D, Augusta de Sa S. Seric ion level and its relationship with the symptoms of premenstrual syndrome in young women. Nutr Hosp. 2013;28(6):2194-2200.

6.      Loria-Kohen V, Gomez-Candela C, Palma-Milla S, Amador-Sastre B, Hernanz A, Bermejo LM. A pilot study of folic acid supplementation for improving homocysteine levels, cognitive and depressive status in eating disorders. Nutr Hosp. 2013;28(3):807-815.

# 15. TOPICAL AGENTS

Pain relievers can be applied directly to your skin. These topical pain relievers are a noninvasive and convenient method for delivering pain-relieving medications. This is especially important and beneficial if you are not able to take medications by mouth. Topical pain relievers include complementary and alternative medications as well as conventional medications. Topical forms of analgesics, or pain relievers, have been used throughout human history.

The use of ointments for medicinal purposes is mentioned in the Bible. The purpose of a topical analgesic is to transmit a medication through your skin into your body. The amount of drug that actually gets through your skin is determined by the amount of pressure applied as you rub it over your skin, the area of your skin covered by the drug, the thickness of your skin and the way in which the drug is dissolved, and the use of dressings over your skin. Analgesics are available in ointments, creams, and gels. They also may be placed in patches that may be applied to your skin.

The advantage of topical analgesics is that they can be placed on your skin over the site of your pain. When compared to oral medications, you will have a lower blood level of the drug and will have fewer side effects and fewer drug interactions. There are different types of topical pain relievers. Ointments are semisolid preparations that melt at body temperature and spread easily. Ointments are not routinely used in the practice of pain medicine unless the ointment is specially compounded by a pharmacy.

Ointments are defined in three categories based on your skin penetration. One type of ointment does not penetrate beyond the external layer of your skin called the epidermis. Ointments of this class can be used for the treatment of sunburn. A second type of ointment penetrates to the internal layer of your skin called the dermis. The third type of ointment actually goes through your skin to the nerves and ligaments and in some instances into your bloodstream. The latter two types of ointments are frequently used in pain management.

Substances applied on your skin can evaporate. You do not want your analgesic drug evaporating from your skin. Your pharmacist will add substances such as glycerin to the ointment to keep this evaporation from happening. Ointments can be prepared by your pharmacist or purchased over the counter or by prescription. Some ointment preparations will contain absorption enhancers. Absorption enhancers make it easier for the drug to be absorbed through your skin. Azone and DMSO can both enhance the absorption of ointments through your skin. Ointments should be packaged in tubes.

Creams are opaque, thick, liquid substances that consist of medications dissolved in a cream base that usually vanishes through the skin. They are less of a liquid consistency than ointments. Gels are a drug-delivery system that usually contain penetration enhancers and are usually used for administering anti-inflammatory medications. The anti-inflammatory medication must be absorbed through your skin to provide you with pain relief. Gels are useful treatment methods if you have arthritic and/or muscle pain. Gels usually are thicker than creams or ointments and are usually clear, unlike creams and ointments.

The concentration of medication in gels is usually no greater than 2 percent. For example, lidocaine, which is a numbing medicine for the control of pain, is dispensed as a 2 percent gel. However, the cream is available in a 5 percent concentration. This is because medications are usually absorbed through the skin better if used in gel form. Gels usually have clarity and sparkle. They maintain their thickness even with an elevated body temperature. Some gels have been developed that may be given nasally. Some drugs are absorbed well through your nose than through your skin. Gels are usually dispensed in tubes or squeeze bottles.

Another delivery system for analgesics is a transdermal patch, which contains medication that is transmitted directly through your skin. A patch containing a medication is placed on your skin and remains there for a specified time so that the drug within the patch can be delivered through your skin to your bloodstream. Local anesthetics such as lidocaine, capsaicin cream, and fentanyl (a potent opioid medication), are some of the medicines that can be delivered through your skin using a transdermal drug delivery system.

Patches should be applied only to areas on your skin that have no blisters or open areas such as a cut. The patches are made of adhesive materials. You should not use the patch if you are allergic to some adhesives. The amount of drug that is absorbed from the patch is directly related to the length of the application of the patch, as well as the area of your skin to which it is applied. The advantage of the patch is that it gives you a continuous flow of analgesic medications.

When you take a pill, after it leaves your stomach or intestine and enters into your bloodstream, you receive a high concentration of the drug initially. As the drug is distributed to other tissues in your body, your blood level concentration of the drug decreases. Once your body breaks down the drug, you will no longer have an analgesic effect of that particular drug. However, when using a patch, you will have a continuous release of the drug from the patch into your bloodstream. You will have constant pain relief without the peaks and valleys of the drug concentration in your bloodstream associated with oral medications.

Natural compounds such as herbs or leaves and roots also can be used to treat your pain topically. Aloe Vera can be used to decrease your pain if you have sunburn. The use of this natural topical product for the treatment of various medical conditions was discovered in 1935. This drug is effective for the treatment of skin inflammation as well as minor burns. Capsaicin is a drug that has been extensively studied in both the clinical and laboratory settings.

Capsaicin is the active component of chili or red peppers. Capsaicin can be placed on your skin over your joints if you have joint pain (osteoarthritis). The capsaicin first stimulates the small pain-transmitting fibers (C fibers) by depleting these fibers of the neurotransmitter substance called P. After the substance P has been depleted, you will have a block of the pain fibers that cause burning pain sensations.

Observations in Hispanic individuals demonstrate that they did not have mouth or stomach pain after ingesting red peppers. The reason is the depletion of the pain-transmitting chemical (substance P) in the nerve endings in these areas following continual exposure to red peppers. Substance P is also present in your joints throughout your body. For this reason, capsaicin can be an effective pain reliever for the treatment of pain associated with osteoarthritis and rheumatoid arthritis. It may take a week for you to feel the pain-relieving effects of capsaicin. As substance P is being depleted from your nerve endings, you nerve endings still manufacture substance P. As a result, it will take several days to deplete enough of the substance P to provide you with pain relief. Once you discontinue use of this cream, your nerves will replenish substance P and your pain may return.

If you have a neuropathy, (e.g. burning foot pain) related to your diabetes you could have significant pain relief with topical capsaicin. Some pain-medicine physicians have used topical capsaicin to relieve the pain associated with shingles. You may have a brief burning sensation following the use of capsaicin. You should be warned to avoid contact with your eyes and genital areas. It is recommended that you use rubber gloves when applying the capsaicin cream. You should use the capsaicin cream no more than three times a day. Various concentrations of capsaicin exist. Begin with a small concentration that contains 0.025 percent capsaicin. You may eventually increase your capsaicin dose to 0.075 percent capsaicin.

Menthol is an oil that is one component of peppermint oil. This oil in a cream base can significantly decrease your pain. When you place a menthol preparation on your skin, the menthol will feel cold to your nerve endings. While you feel the cold, your pain-stimulating nerves will be depressed. Following the initial cool sensation, you will feel a period of warmth. Menthol products can be used for the treatment of pain associated with arthritis, muscle pain, and tendonitis. Application of a menthol-containing cream may be of benefit to you if you suffer from tension headaches. It can be rubbed around the neck muscles just below the skull. It can be an extremely effective method for the treatment of your headaches.

Allergic reactions with menthol have been reported. It is recommended that you test a small amount of menthol on your skin before applying it extensively to assure yourself that you are not allergic it. You should not use the menthol preparation more than three times a day. Do not use a heating pad or a cold pack over the area of your skin where the menthol substance was placed. Some natural herbs and vegetable juices can be used as topical analgesics as well. One example is onion juice.

It is reported by some doctors that spreading the juice of a sliced onion over one of your painful areas could reduce your pain. A tincture can be made by putting 100 grams of minced onions in 30 grams of ethanol for a 70 percent solution. There are no hazards or side effects associated with the topical administration of an onion. However, frequent contact with the onion over time could possibly lead to an allergic reaction. The bark of a poplar tree also can be used for relieving your pain. The bark can be used for control of your pain over your joints or nerves or if you have rheumatoid arthritis. You should not use the bark if you are allergic to aspirin.

When externally applied to painful areas of your skin using the poplar bark and leaves, you should use no more than five grams of the drug per day. Either when using these topical natural products, you must follow the directions for the use of these medicines that are contained on the outside of the package or from an insert that may be placed in a box that holds a tube of any of these substances. You should remember that although these are natural products, they could have side effects like any other medication.

Another topical medication used to prevent pain is EMLA cream. This cream is dispensed only by prescription. It is used as a numbing agent more than it is used for reducing pain. This is a cream consisting of lidocaine and prilocaine, which are both numbing agents. This local anesthetic combination is packaged in tubes. An EMLA cellulose disc can be applied over your painful area. The purpose of EMLA is to provide pain relief over the painful area of your skin. It is used in children to reduce the pain of starting intravenous lines. Some pain-management doctors advocate its use to decrease the pain associated with reflex sympathetic dystrophy or the pain associated with shingles. This cream should be placed on an intact skin area.

The EMLA should be applied under a bandage for at least 60 minutes to provide relief over the painful area of your skin. This cream is not recommended if you have an allergy to lidocaine or prilocaine. If you have the blood disorder called methemoglobinemia, you should not use this cream. You should not exceed the recommended dose prescribed by your physician.

The problem with this cream as opposed to the Lidoderm patches is that it does provide pain relief for your skin but it can also numb your skin. This could be a problem if your skin becomes numb. This means that you have a block of all sensation in the skin treated with this cream. You should avoid causing any trauma to the area, including scratching your skin or rubbing or exposing your skin to extreme hot or cold temperatures until you have complete return of sensation to your skin. It is recommended that you not use this medication if you are taking heart medication. The local anesthetics in this cream can interact with some heart medicines.

Another analgesic cream that is available over the counter is a combination of methyl salicylate and menthol. This is a cream that is effective for the temporary relief of arthritis and pain in your muscles. You should not use this medicine if your skin is sensitive to the oil of wintergreen. You should apply this cream around the sore areas on your body. You should not apply this cream more than three times a day. Do not place this cream over areas of the skin that are broken

Steroid creams are sometimes used for the treatment of joint pain. Topical steroids are anti-inflammatory agents. Pramoxine hydrochloride is a topical anesthetic agent that sometimes is combined with steroids to attempt to manage pain. This cream provides a temporary relief from pain. You should not use this cream if you are allergic to any of the substances in the cream such as the steroid or the pramoxine. If you develop a rash or blistering, you must stop using the cream. You should not use this cream more than three times a day. Furthermore, do not use this steroid preparation for more than five days. Do not reuse this cream until you have discussed the situation with your doctor.

Nonsteroidal anti-inflammatory agents (NSAIDS) may be compounded into creams by your pharmacist. These creams should not be used more than three times a day. Side effects with the nonsteroidal anti-inflammatory creams are the same as with the NSAIDs taken by mouth. However, the side effects of the topical NSAIDS are less than the oral

NSAIDS. The side effects of any NSAID can include stomach upset and allergic reactions. If the dose is high enough, it could affect both your liver and kidneys. These NSAIDs can be very effective for the management of your pain when applied over your skin.

The use of a ketoprofen gel and a diclofenac gel, both NSAIDs, were compared at painful sites in a four-week study. The ketoprofen gel gave positive results for the treatment of knee pain and was shown to be better at relieving pain than the diclofenac gel. If you have joint pain, you may want to discuss these facts with your pain-medicine doctor or orthopedic doctor. Aspirin creams also may provide you with some pain relief when applied over your painful joints or muscles. Amitriptyline and ketamine are prescription drugs that may be mixed together to provide pain relief.

Ketamine is a potent analgesic that requires a prescription. Ketamine is a medication that can cause you to hallucinate if the dose is too high. A high dose of Ketamine is similar to LSD in its pharmacological effects. Elavil, an antidepressant can be applied topically to provide you with pain relief. A study in animals has used both of these agents together to treat pain in the laboratory setting. Amitriptyline, which is an antidepressant, has recently been shown to have pain-relieving properties when applied topically. Amitriptyline cream may be advantageous if you do not want to take amitriptyline pills by mouth.

An amitriptyline cream will not help you if you are suffering from significant depression, but can be helpful in decreasing your pain. Some patients complain of being tired while taking amitriptyline. However, amitriptyline can contribute to pain relief in fibromyalgia and the topical application may be a way of avoiding significant side effects that can be associated with oral use. There is ongoing research in this area. You may want to keep informed of the research on both of these drugs through the National Library of Medicine website at www.nlm.nih.gov.

The transdermal fentanyl patch system has become popular since it was introduced in the 1980s. This strong opioid medication was used initially for cancer pain management and then for noncancerous, chronic pain management. Fentanyl is able penetrate your skin easily. Fentanyl is 75 times more potent than morphine. It produces less histamine release from cells in your bloodstream and causes less itching than morphine. The fentanyl patch is primarily used for chronic or cancer-related pain.

A fentanyl patch can be used for most moderate to severe pain syndromes. In the fentanyl patch, the medication exists as a gel in a drug reservoir. Between this reservoir and your skin is a release membrane that has various-size holes that regulate the amount of fentanyl that is delivered to your skin. The larger the size of the holes will allow more fentanyl to be distributed to your skin and eventually through your skin which gives you a higher dose of the drug. The adhesiveness around the patch keeps it in place.

When the fentanyl patch is placed on your skin the fentanyl diffuses through the holes in the release membrane to the surface of your skin. It then goes to the outer layer of your skin and is deposited in a storage area. From the storage area, it is gradually absorbed into your blood-stream. This is the reason that it takes at least an hour before the fentanyl has begun to enter your bloodstream.

You will probably not notice any pain-relieving effects from this drug delivery system for about six hours. The patch is usually removed every three days. After the patch is removed, you will still have some drug that remains in the storage area under your skin. If you remove the patch and do not replace it, you will still receive fentanyl for hours after the patch has been removed.

Fentanyl patches come in different concentrations. The concentrations correlate with the area of the skin to which they are applied. The effectiveness of the patch is not affected by placing it on your chest, your back, or your upper arm. An increase in temperature will cause the medication to be rapidly delivered from the patch to your bloodstream.

Your skin's thickness also can affect the amount of fentanyl that is absorbed through your skin. The thicker your skin, the slower the rate of delivery of the fentanyl will be. The patch should not be applied over broken skin because the blood level of fentanyl can be significantly raised. There is no barrier to slow the absorption of the fentanyl. The fentanyl patch can cause a decrease in breathing and even death if you receive a significantly high dose of the fentanyl.

Occasionally, you may require medication for breakthrough pain if you do something to aggravate your chronic pain syndrome. For example, if you are using the patch for chronic pain and you go into your garden and do lifting, pushing, or digging, you may cause the onset of temporary pain on top of your chronic pain. At that time, an oral medication can be taken for treatment of your breakthrough pain. Another popular patch that is readily available by prescription from your pain-management doctor is the lidocaine-containing patch called Lidoderm.

The Lidoderm transdermal drug-delivery system exerts a significant amount of its pain-relieving effects by releasing a small amount of lidocaine into your bloodstream. Lidocaine is a local anesthetic. The patch does not cause numbness over your skin but does give you some degree of pain relief below the patch. There also is an effect on the nerves under your skin that are transmitting pain. This patch is used for the treatment of shingles. The Lidoderm patch contains 5 percent lidocaine. The lidocaine essentially does not reach your bloodstream like fentanyl.

The lidocaine penetrates your skin just enough to reach the nerve endings that are transmitting your pain. As a result, there are minimal side effects from the use of this patch other than from the adhesive layer of the patch. The amount of the lidocaine that is absorbed from the Lidoderm is related to the length of application over your skin. The patch should be used for 12 hours over your painful area and then removed for 12 hours. If an irritation or a burning sensation occurs around the adhesive aspect of the patch, you should discontinue use of the patch. None of the patches mentioned in this chapter should ever be reused.

You must be aware that the Lidoderm patch does contain methyl paraben, which is found in many suntan lotions. Do not use the Lidoderm patch if you have allergies to any suntan lotions that contain this chemical. You should not use the Lidoderm patch if you are using a heart drug to control your heartbeat. Even though the amount of lidocaine that you can absorb is small, it can interfere with some heart medicines. If you are using heart medications, discuss any potential drug interactions with you doctor. If you become lightheaded following application of the patch, you must stop using the patch immediately.

Clonidine is another transdermal medication (Catepress). This patch is applied weekly to one area of your skin. The clonidine patch inhibits the release of norepinephrine, which is a pain transmitter. The clonidine patch also is used for the treatment of hypertension. If you have neuropathic (nerve injury) pain or reflex sympathetic dystrophy, the clonidine patch may provide you with significant pain relief. It also can be successfully used if you have pain following shingles.

The application of the clonidine patch can be most useful for pain associated with a nerve injury or inflammation of a nerve. The clonidine patch will not completely relieve your pain if you have reflex sympathetic dystrophy or post-shingles pain, but it can significantly decrease the burning component of your pain. The patch comes in different doses. The usual dose is the 0.1-milligram patch that is applied weekly.

Given that no two people are alike, if you are taking any medications and begin to take nutritional supplements you should be aware that potential drug-nutrient interactions may occur and are encouraged to consult a health care professional before using any natural product. Combining certain prescription drugs and dietary supplements can lead to undesirable effects such as: diminished prescription drug effectiveness, reduced supplement effectiveness and impaired drug and/or supplement absorption.

The plant polyphenol, resveratrol, naturally occurring in a number of fruits and other food products, has been extensively studied over the last two decades for its beneficial properties. Recently, its possible topical use in ameliorating skin conditions has also been proposed. The topical use of resveratrol can provide a good defense against induced skin damaged pain.[1]

Experiments have shown that soybean-germ oil (SGO) possesses a remarkable protective activity against UVB-induced skin inflammation. These results suggest that SGO might have interesting therapeutic and cosmetic applications in the management of some painful skin diseases initiated, sustained, or exacerbated by an over production of free radicals.[2]

The effect of dietary supplements based on Resveratrol, Lycopene, Vitamin C and Anthocyanins in reducing skin toxicity pain due to external beam radiotherapy in patients affected by breast cancer has been reported as well.[3]

References

1.     Sticozzi C, Cervellati F, Muresan XM, Cervellati C, Valacchi G. Resveratrol prevents cigarette smoke-induced keratinocytes damage. Food Funct. 2014;5(9):2348-2356.

2.     Bonina F, Puglia C, Avogadro M, Baranelli E, Cravotto G. The topical protective effect of soybean-germ oil against UVB-induced cutaneous erythema: an in vivo evaluation. Arch Pharm (Weinheim). 2005;338(12):598-601.

3.     Di Franco R, Calvanese M, Murino P, et al. Skin toxicity from external beam radiation therapy in breast cancer patients: protective effects of Resveratrol, Lycopene, Vitamin C and anthocianin (Ixor(R)). Radiat Oncol. 2012;7:12.

# 16. ALTERNATIVE THERAPIES

Alternative medicine may be very effective in decreasing your pain. Many conventional medicine pain practices include alternative medicine clinicians as part of their multidisciplinary treatment. For example practices include alternative medicine clinicians as part of their multidisciplinary treatment. For example, acupuncture may be offered in some pain practices. "Conventional medicine" is practiced by medical doctors (M.D.) or doctors of osteopathy (D.O.).

Conventional medicine includes methods practiced by allied health-care professionals such as physical therapists, occupational therapists, psychologists, and registered nurses. Other terms for conventional medicine include allopathic medicine, mainstream medicine, and orthodox medicine.

Complementary and alternative medicine is referred to as unconventional or non-conventional medicine. The following is a definition for alternative medicine specialties by the National Center for Complementary and Alternative Medicine. "Complementary and alternative medicines are practices and products that are not currently considered to be part of conventional medicine." Complementary and alternative medicine practices change and update continually.

The National Institute of Health (NIH) is reviewing alternative therapies and is confirming efficacy and safety in some areas. Complementary and alternative medicines, unlike many conventional medicine therapies, are designed to help you develop control over your health. If you are going to use any of these methods, you are encouraged to learn the side effects of some of these medicines as well as learn about drug interactions with conventional medications.

These interactions can be lethal. Do not be afraid to tell your physician what complementary medicines you are taking. Remember that when you are using alternative medicines that these medicines are not strictly controlled with respect to dosage and the amount of drug in a pill, capsule, or tea.

All plants have different amounts of substances in them. A true dose of an alternative medication in a pill is unknown in many instances. You should look carefully at the label before taking one of these substances and not take more than the label recommends. The overall drug interactions of herbal substances have not been established because they are not required to be studied by the FDA.

Conventional medical professionals are beginning to recognize the benefits of alternative medicine. As an example, the National Institute of Health Office of Alternative Medicine was established in 1992. In addition, there has been a significant increase in professional interest in the area of alternative medicine. Medical schools are beginning to offer elective courses on alternative medical therapies. The attitudes of medical school faculty toward the use of complementary medicine practices are important because the attitude of these individuals can influence their students.

Some health plans have now announced their intention to incorporate payment for some alternative medicine practices into their insurance coverage. Some managed care corporations have revealed their intentions to include alternative medicine practices for payment. Some state governments are considering legislation pertaining to the practice of alternative medicine by health-care professionals.

If you are going to use a natural substance or therapy, you are responsible for your own care. You must not self-diagnose yourself. You must discuss your symptoms of pain with your physician before taking any nutritional supplement. Grapefruit juice taken for weight loss for example may decrease the absorption of some medications from your stomach. As a result, you may not be getting the medicine that you need.

There are risks and benefits that you should be aware of when using alternative medications and therapies to manage your pain. In addition, the alternative medications you take could react with the prescription medications your doctor has given you and cause you even more problems. For example, high doses of vitamin E can decrease your blood's ability to form a blood clot.

If you are taking a blood thinner like Plavix in addition to vitamin E, you could develop a serious bleeding problem. If in doubt, consult the Physician's Drug Reference for herbal medicines. This will advise you about safe doses and any precautions and drug interactions that you may need to be aware of.

There was a study published in the New England Journal of Medicine in 1993 that was a survey of individuals in order to get their opinion of alternative medicine practices. More than 30 percent of those surveyed at that time chose alternative medicine over conventional medicine methods to prevent and treat disease.

In 1994, Congress passed the Dietary Supplement Health and Education Act. In passing this act, Congress recognized that many individuals believed that dietary supplements offered health benefits. The bill gave dietary supplement manufacturers freedom to produce more products and to provide information about their products' health benefits. The Food and Drug Administration (FDA), on the other hand, is responsible for overseeing any claims by the dietary supplement The FDA monitors manufacturers to the truthfulness of their claims.

The Federal Trade Commission regulates the advertising of all of the dietary supplements. You should be aware that the quality control standards for natural substances are a problem within this industry. Some of the manufacturers of these products will not have the amount of substance in the natural medication as stated on the container label.

You need to know that when you are using alternative medicines that these medicines are not strictly controlled with respect to dosage and the amount of drug in a pill, capsule, or tea. All plants have different amounts of chemicals in them. A true dose of a medication is unknown in many instances. You should look carefully at the label before taking one of these substances and not take more than the label recommends.

The overall drug interactions of herbal substances have not been established because they are not required to be studied by the FDA. You must do your own research to determine whether the natural substance that you are taking has an accurate dosage as stated on the container label for the product.

Alternative medicine is now recognized as a legitimate medical practice. Many physicians have had personal experience with alternative medicines and felt that they were effective. Before treatment by an alternative medicine specialist, inquire to ascertain that they are properly trained. In other words, inquire as to whether or not that they have had training in alternative medicine science.

For example if you want acupuncture, you should inquire if there are state requirements for the practice of acupuncture. Someone that is not trained could cause you harm. The NIH does award grants for the study of research in complementary as well as alternative medicines. Clinical trials are being done throughout the United States with respect to complementary and alternative medicines. You may want to participate in one of these trials.

Study trials with respect to herbal medicines are an important part of the medical research process. The results from clinical trials can define better ways to treat your painful conditions. A clinical trial is a research study in which a therapy is tested on individuals like you to ensure that the medicine being tested is safe and effective. Always remember that clinical trials have risks. Before participating in a clinical trial, discuss this trial with your primary care physician. To find out about ongoing clinical trials for example, studies on arthritis and neurological disorders go to www.nccam.nih.gov.

You also may want to access the National Library of Medicine online (www.pubmed.com). Complementary medicine on PubMed is available that contains citations to articles on recently published research. You may want to see a homeopathic or naturopathic specialist. Homeopathic specialists prescribe dilutions of natural substances from plants, minerals, and animals. Homeopathy has been around for more than 200 years.

About 500 million people around the world receive homeopathic treatment. The World Health Organization has recommended that homeopathy is a system of traditional medicine that should be integrated with conventional medicine, which is considered the traditional approach to medicine.

It is important to know that the U.S. Food and Drug Administration recognizes homeopathic remedies as official drugs and regulates their manufacture. This is unlike the herbs used for medicinal use. Conventional physicians in Europe use homeopathy qualities of medicine frequently. In Britain, homeopathy is a part of the national health system.

The basic principles of homeopathy are that a disease can be destroyed and removed by a type of medicine that is able to produce the disease in humans. In other words, a substance that in large doses would produce symptoms of a disease can be used in very minute doses to cure it. In conventional medicine, this is called the theory of antibiotics.

Homeopathic practitioners adhere to the fact that the more a substance is diluted, the more potent it is. In conventional medicine, it is believed that a higher dose of the medicine will lead to a greater effect. The purpose of diluting out substances in homeopathic medicine is to avoid side effects. Homeopathic practitioners adhere to the fact that illness is different for every person. Homeopathic treatments are unique for each patient.

Homeopathic medicine emphasizes that patients are individuals and have individual signs and symptoms of an illness and should be treated only on an individual basis. The entire individual is treated, which includes the physical, psychological and spiritual portions of each person. Naturopathic medicine treats disease by using your body's natural ability to heal itself. Naturopathic practitioners invoke healing processes by using a variety of treatment options based on your particular needs. In naturopathic medicine, disease symptoms are a sign of your body's attempt to heal itself.

The steroid can be given over approximately two weeks. Sometimes your doctor will inject your painful joint with a steroid. Colchicine is the medication that has been used extensively over the past two decades for the treatment of gout. It is most effective during the first 24 hours of an acute attack. Colchicine can cause you to have vomiting and nausea. If you have liver problems, you should not take colchicine.

Allopurinol is another drug that can decrease your uric acid levels. Allopurinol is usually used in people who produce excessive uric acid. Allopurinol should not be used during an acute gouty arthritis episode because Allopurinol can prolong the attack. Some rheumatologists prescribe probenecid because it has fewer side effects than Allopurinol. Some patients may need narcotics for management of their pain.

If you have developed tophi (nodules under your skin) that are painful, you may need to have these uric acid crystals removed surgically. If you have had significant destruction of one of your joints, an orthopedic surgeon may need to surgically correct any malformation that may be related to uric acid deposition in your joints and the resultant joint naturally. Naturopathic medicine gets its data from Chinese, Native American, and Greek cultures.

Reflexology is another method used in nonconventional medicine practice to decrease your pain. Reflexology relieves muscle stress and relaxes your muscles through the application of pressure on specific areas of your feet. Reflexology has been used for thousands of years in mideastern countries. In the early twentieth century, a doctor mapped the foot areas that related to areas of the body that affected different medical conditions.

This doctor divided the body into 10 zones and he labeled parts of the foot that he believed controlled each zone. Gentle pressure on an area of the foot would generate not only pain relief but healing in general in the defined zone. These areas of pressure in your feet are called reflex points.

The philosophy of reflexology is that your body contains an energy field. When your energy field is blocked, you develop pain and/or illness. Stimulation of your foot and the nerves that end in your feet can unblock the energy flow and increase energy to various parts of your body and promote healing as well as decrease your pain. It also is believed that stimulation of your feet can release the natural painkillers in your body called endorphins. Reflexology treatment sessions can last from 30 to 60 minutes. Usually you will receive a four-week treatment program.

Reflexology can be used for the management of your back pain. Reflexologists believe that nerve endings in the feet have inner connection throughout the spinal cord and brain to reach all areas of the body. The problem with reflexology is that it has not been scientifically studied and still remains an unproven treatment regimen for the management of your pain.

A therapeutic massage can significantly help you control your pain, especially if you have muscle spasms. Massage therapy can decrease your stress as well as decrease your headaches and pain associated with whiplash injuries.

Massage therapy promotes generalized body relaxation. Massage is the application of touch to your muscles or ligaments that does not cause you to move or change position of a joint. Massage therapy can decrease your lower back pain as well as your neck pain. It also has been effective to reduce pain associated with sciatica. Massage therapy can decrease the pain associated with tension headaches.

There are different types of massage therapy. The Swedish massage is the most common form of massage therapy in the United States. Swedish massage works on the superficial layers of the skin as well as the superficial muscles of your body. Swedish massage promotes relaxation and improves circulation in your superficial muscles. Another type of massage is deep-tissue massage. This is more direct pressure on the deeper muscle layers of your body.

Deep-tissue massage is highly effective for the treatment of lower back pain. Sports massage combines Swedish massage with deep-tissue massage. This type of massage therapy can decrease your pain following a vigorous athletic workout. It may not be a good idea to use therapeutic massage if you have certain forms of cancer, heart disease, or some infectious diseases.

Another method to help you control your pain is aromatherapy. Women have a better perception of smell than men. Therefore, women are more likely to use aromatherapy because they have better results from this method than men.

For hundreds of years, oils extracted from plants have been used to relieve pain. During your first session with an aromatherapy specialist, the specialist will select the oil that is appropriate for relieving your pain. You may have a treatment for up to nine minutes.

Aromatherapy stimulates pleasure centers in your brain from nerves in the nose that senses smell. Aromatherapy can be used to improve your quality of life and provide you with some relaxation. It has been used for pain management during childbirth. It can be used if you have arthritis, back pain, neck pain, and other chronic pain syndromes.

Aromatherapy is reportedly effective for the treatment of muscle pain as well as pain that originates from a nerve injury. You must not use any of the aromatherapy oils if you are allergic to the herbs from which the oils were derived. If you have trouble breathing, you should not use aromatherapy. Some aromatherapy can cause drowsiness.

Sage, rosemary, and juniper oils may increase uterine contractions if you are pregnant. You should not use these oils during pregnancy. Essential oils such as clove, cinnamon, and thyme can have anti-inflammatory properties and are useful in decreasing your joint pain if you have arthritis. Aromatherapy can be used in the following preparations: nose drops, air sprays, steam tents, candles, and drops in your bath.

Acupuncture is another popular method that can be used for pain management. Acupuncture can decrease both your pain as well as your stress. Acupuncture originated in China more than 2,000 years ago. Acupuncture is based on the belief that your health is determined by a balanced flow of vital life energy referred to as chi.

There are 12 major energy pathways in your body called meridians. Each meridian is linked to a specific internal organ. There are more than 1,000 acupoints within the meridians of your body. Stimulation of these meridians enhances the flow of your vital life energy.

Needles are inserted just under your skin to stimulate these meridians and provide you with pain relief. It is believed that acupuncture releases the body's own chemicals that relieve pain, called endorphins and enkephlins. These two chemicals are your body's natural pain-killing chemicals. Acupuncture can decrease the production as well as the distribution of substances that cause pain nerve impulses to go to the brain. Acupuncture, therefore, can decrease your need for conventional pain pills. Acupuncture has been demonstrated to decrease muscle-tension headaches.

In 1997, the National Institutes of Health endorsed acupuncture for postoperative pain, dental pain, tennis elbow, and carpal tunnel syndrome. The World Health Organization has reported that acupuncture can be useful for the treatment of migraine headaches, trigeminal neuralgia, sciatica, and arthritis.

Acupuncture also can be used to treat fibromyalgia, neck pain, and back pain. In some states there is no licensing required to be an acupuncturist, whereas other states limit the practice to medical doctors and chiropractors. In some states acupuncturists are considered primary health-care professionals and may see you without your doctor's referral.

Some states require that an acupuncturist graduate from an approved school and pass a state licensing examination. To find physicians that practice acupuncture, you can go to the website www.medicalacupuncture.org. Furthermore, the American Association of Oriental Medicine has a website, www.aaom.org, which is a national trade organization of acupuncturists who have met acceptable standards of competency. This organization can provide you with the names and locations of competent members of this organization in your community.

Naturopaths recommend healing of the person and not the disease. Naturopathic medicinal treatments will include doses of natural substances that are much higher than those used by practitioners of homeopathic medicine. To best choose a natural product to decrease your pain, you should know which chemicals in the body produce pain. With this knowledge, you can pick the analgesic best suited to relieve your pain. If you have joint pain, for instance, you will want to use an alternative medicine that has anti-inflammatory properties.

If you are injured or have inflammation, your body makes a variety of chemicals that transmit pain impulses to a pain-processing center in your brain. These chemicals include the prostaglandins, cytokines, substance P, glutamic acid, and nitric oxide. Nitric oxide is a gas that is a pain chemical transmitter in your nervous system. Some remedies will be mentioned in this chapter. For in depth information, it is recommended that you consult a naturopathic book.

Given that no two people are alike, if you are taking any medications and begin to take nutritional supplements you should be aware that potential drug-nutrient interactions may occur and are encouraged to consult a health care professional before using any natural product. Combining certain prescription drugs and dietary supplements can lead to undesirable effects such as: diminished prescription drug effectiveness, reduced supplement effectiveness and impaired drug and/or supplement absorption.

The spice, turmeric has anti-inflammatory and antioxidant effects and has been shown to inhibit prostaglandin formation. This drug should not be used if you have gallbladder disease. Furthermore, do not use this medicine if you have hypertension. No significant serious health risks or side effects with use of this substance have been reported to date. The average dose is 3 grams of turmeric per day. This dose can be divided up into 1-gram doses and be taken 3 times per day with meals. For example, you may take 1 milligram with each meal for a total dose of 3 grams.

Ginseng has anti-inflammatory effects and is used in homeopathic medicine for the treatment of rheumatoid arthritis. Do not use ginseng with caffeine. Exercise caution if you use ginseng along with any antidiabetic medicine or insulin. You should not use ginseng with MAOI inhibitors, which are used to decrease your blood pressure.

Do not use ginseng in combination with diuretics. Side effects include sleep deprivation, nosebleeds, headaches, nervousness, and vomiting.

The average daily dose of this root is 1 to 2 grams. Do not take more than 2 grams per day. The 2 grams can be divided up and taken 3 times a day.

Resveratrol is an antioxidant and a COX-2 inhibitor that some believe prevents heart disease and cancer. It is largely found in the skin of red grapes. Therefore, many people obtain resveratrol by drinking red wine. This substance can prevent clot formation, whereas the conventional COX-2 inhibitors do not prevent clot formation. The usual dose is no more than 600 mg per day. There are no known side effects or drug interactions for resveratrol itself. Fish oils contain the omega-3 fatty acids and can decrease prostaglandins.

Fish oils are used for the treatment of rheumatoid arthritis. You also may use fish oils for the control of joint pain. The most common side effect that you may experience with fish oil supplementation is mild stomach upset. The fish oils can decrease your blood's ability to clot. If you are taking blood-thinning drugs, you should not take fish oils, because it will give you an increased risk of bleeding. You may take up to 10 grams of fish oil per day.

N-acetylcysteine is an amino acid produced by your body that will decrease prostaglandin formation. It can help prevent some diseases and boost your immune system. You should not take this drug if you are taking carbamazepine (Tegretol). Side effects include headaches, nausea, vomiting, and an upset stomach. The recommended dose is 200 milligrams 3 times a day.

Cayenne is an anti-inflammatory medication that is helpful for the treatment of muscle pain and arthritis. This drug may be helpful for inhibiting the release of substance P (a pain signal transmitter) as well. Cayenne side effects include diarrhea and intestinal colic. It can decrease your body's ability to form a normal blood clot. It also can reduce the effects of aspirin, so you should be aware of this fact if you are taking aspirin as a blood thinner. High doses of cayenne over a prolonged time can cause kidney and liver damage. You should not use this drug for more than two days in a row. After two weeks you may use it again for two days. The daily dose of cayenne should not exceed 10 grams.

Ipriflavone can be used as a prostaglandin inhibitor. Women also use it to decrease the incidence of osteoporosis. This medicine can actually stop bone loss. It can decrease the risk of fractures in bone pain in females. This drug, like the other drugs that are prostaglandin inhibitors, can increase the blood-thinning activity of other drugs that you may be taking, such as Coumadin. It also can increase the effects of some asthma drugs such as theophylline, so avoid taking ipriflavone if you are using such medications.

Procyanidolic oligomers are natural substances extracted from grape seeds. They are useful for their antioxidant effects. They can decrease arthritis pain. There are no significant side effects associated with this drug. The daily dose of this drug ranges from 150 to 300 milligrams per day. However, another important effect of this medicine is that it can decrease the effects of nitric oxide.

Nitric oxide is sometimes released from cells in your bloodstream. Nitric acid essentially exists in a gas form in your body and this gas stimulates pain fibers to transmit pain impulses to your brain. Nitric oxide inhibitors include the fish oils. Cytokines are chemicals produced in your bloodstream that also enhance pain impulses. They contribute to the formation of substances that can destroy your joint linings if you have rheumatoid arthritis. Fish oils can reduce these substances in your body. These are just some examples of natural substances that can help you control your chronic pain.

Increased recognition of the limits of conventional medicine has helped drive the growing interest in complementary and alternative medicine which is now being commonly used in patients with chronic diseases, including individuals with Crohn's disease and ulcerative colitis.[1]

Alternative and complementary therapeutic approaches, such as the use of a wide array of herbal, nutritional, and physical manipulations, are becoming popular for relieving symptoms of osteoarthritis (OA). There is evidence of possible beneficial effects of SP in the management of OA.[2]

References

1.      Ali T, Shakir F, Morton J. Curcumin and inflammatory bowel disease: biological mechanisms and clinical implication. Digestion. 2012;85(4):249-255.

2.      Arjmandi BH, Khalil DA, Lucas EA, et al. Soy protein may alleviate osteoarthritis symptoms. Phytomedicine. 2004;11(7-8):567-575.

# 17. CHIROPRACTIC THERAPY

Chiropractic therapy was established as a profession in 1895. It is now the second-largest primary health-care field in the world. You may be scared of the dangers and side effects of pills and procedures that may lead you to seek out chiropractic therapy. Chiropractic therapy as a profession emphasizes your body's natural health abilities. Many people associate chiropractic therapy with only back and neck pain. However, chiropractic therapy has been shown to be safe for the treatment of headaches, carpal tunnel syndrome, and pain in your arms and legs.

Low back pain may have many causes. In most cases of injury or strain it takes time for your back to heal. Back pain lasts just as long if you go to a chiropractor, if you go to a physical therapist or if you seek no treatment at all. Chiropractic manipulationand conventional medical care are about equally effective for relieving acute low back pain. Chiropractic treatment is based on the concept that restricted movement in the spine may lead to pain and reduced function.

Spinal adjustment is just one form of therapy chiropractors use to treat restricted spinal mobility. During an adjustment, chiropractors use their hands to apply a controlled, sudden force to a joint. Chiropractors may also use massage and stretching to relax muscles that are shortened or in spasm. Many use additional treatments as well, such as ultrasound, electrical muscle stimulation and exercises.

Chiropractic medicine can improve your body function and enhance your body's healing powers. Some chiropractors emphasize a healthful lifestyle, a healthful diet, and stress reduction. They will educate you with respect to your lifestyle at each visit. Many times you doctor will refer you to a chiropractor or physical therapist if you have neck and back pain. In many instances your doctor will refer you to a chiropractor, who often works together with a physical therapist working at their clinic. Both of these professions can help you with your chronic pain.

The definition of chiropractic therapy is the correction of problems that exist in your spinal column. This enables your body to function at its peak level without medications, surgical procedures, or steroid injections. In 1999, more than 25 million Americans were treated by chiropractors. Not only do chiropractors take care of back injuries, they also can help you with your neck, hip, leg, ankle, foot, arm, and hand pain. Most back and neck pains are the result of mechanical disorders in your spine.

The problem with chiropractic medicine is that it has been maligned for a long time in the United States. However, it is now widely accepted. In Canada, which is under a national health-care system, chiropractic care is included among treatment methods that are reimbursed by the national system. If you have a back injury caused by a twist or turn, you may want to go to a chiropractor. If you have a back injury and need strengthening exercises, your doctor may refer you to a physical therapist.

Chiropractic medicine focuses attention on the relationship between the structure of your spine and how it affects your nervous system. If your spine is not in alignment due to slouching or poor posture, this can cause some of your nerves to be compressed by your spine. Your chiropractor will adjust your spine to remove any spinal abnormalities to reduce pressure off of the nerves in your arms and legs.

When your spine is not aligned correctly, it can cause you to experience tension in your muscles that will in turn affect your nervous system (spinal cord and the nerves emerging from your spinal cord). Compression on your spine and the nerves that come off of your spinal cord can cause you significant health problems and pain. In many instances an adjustment of your spine can remedy these problems.

Following your initial care, your chiropractor may re-evaluate your progress from time to time. After your spine has been misaligned for any length of time, your body may have a tendency to resume that misalignment again. Therefore, periodic visits with your chiropractor are recommended.

Traction is another method that is frequently used by chiropractors and physical therapists and can be an effective treatment for back pain. Traction involves mechanical forces that separate adjacent body parts away from each other. If you have problems with a disc in your neck or back, traction can separate the bones in your back and increase your blood flow to your injured disc, which can speed up the healing process.

If traction worsens of your pain, you should inform your health-care provider so that the traction can be immediately discontinued. Because of the differences in muscle mass between men and women, the amount of traction applied will differ between men and women. If you have a ruptured disc in your neck or back, traction can help heal this painful entity.

Chiropractors treat other entities besides back pain. For example, if you have a carpal tunnel syndrome, chiropractic manipulation can sometimes correct this condition. On occasion, you may not need surgery after chiropractic treatment.

Given that no two people are alike, if you are taking any medications and begin to take nutritional supplements you should be aware that potential drug-nutrient interactions may occur and are encouraged to consult a health care professional before using any natural product. Combining certain prescription drugs and dietary supplements can lead to undesirable effects such as: diminished prescription drug effectiveness, reduced supplement effectiveness and impaired drug and/or supplement absorption.

Chiropractic and nutritional treatment contribute to the amelioration and perhaps reversal of osteoarthritis (OA). It is further proposed that the chiropractic manipulative thrust, is in effect, treating dysfunctional bio-mechanics of joints, affecting positive cartilaginous change. The pathophysi-ology and multi-factorial causes of OA are reviewed. New interpretations of the literature surrounding OA are discussed which offer arguments for OA's treatment and reversal through chiropractic manipulation and nutrutional support.[1]

Reference

1.      Berkson DL. Osteoarthritis, chiropractic, and nutrition: oste-oarthritis considered as a natural part of a three stage subluxation complex: its reversibility: its relevance and treatability by chiropractic and nutritional correlates. Med Hypotheses. 1991;36(4):356-367.

Psychological factors such as your mood, beliefs about your pain and your coping style have been found to play important roles in your adjustment to chronic pain. For example, if your pain persists over time, you may avoid doing regular activities for fear of further injury or increased pain. This can include work, social activities, or hobbies. As you withdraw and become less active, your muscles may become weaker, you may begin to gain or lose weight, and your overall physical conditioning may decline. Nutrition on the other hand may help your mood.

If your pain persists, you may feel that your pain will never get better. You may then become anxious or depressed. These types of thoughts, along with decreased participation in enjoyable and reinforcing activities, can cause depression and anxiety. The fact that psychological have an impact on your experience of pain does not mean that the pain is in your head or is not real. Most people who report pain are really experiencing it, even if a physical cause cannot be identified.

As you can see, your mind can influence your pain. For example, if you are anxious and depressed you experience of pain becomes worse. On the other hand severe pain can cause anxiety and depression. Chronic pain can impact all areas of your life and is often associated with functional, psychological and social problems.

Psychological factors such as mood, beliefs about pain and coping style have been found to play an important role in your adjustment to your chronic pain. For example you may avoid doing regular activities for fear of further injury or increased pain. This can include work, social activities, or hobbies.

Psychological problems can contribute to the belief that one is disabled. As pain persists, you may develop negative beliefs about your pain. These thoughts may make you feel depressed and anxious. The fact that psychological factors can have an impact on your experience of pain does not mean that the pain is not real. Remember that pain is an unpleasant sensory and emotional response to tissue trauma. Your doctor may refer you for a psychological evaluation.

You will be required to describe your pain to your psychologist. These tests were described in more detail in a previous chapter. Using descriptive words is one method of describing your pain. A pain-rating index consists of groups of words associated with pain. This index has been incorporated into the McGill pain questionnaire, a type of verbal assessment that uses word descriptors that are valuable in discriminating between different pain syndromes. An example of clinical behavioral medicine is the treatment of chronic pain by "unlearning" it. Some people suffer injuries, resulting in pain and disability, but after they heal physically the pain remains.

A McGill pain questionnaire is a method for assessing pain psychologically. A McGill pain questionnaire gives a multidimensional pain score. You are given 20 word sets that describe a different dimension of your pain. You are asked to select words relevant to your pain from each of these 20 sets. For example, one set includes the words "jumping," "flashing," and "shooting." Another set includes the words "tingling," "itching," "smarting," and "stinging." You circle the word that relates closest to the pain you feel throughout the 20 word sets.

This questionnaire is difficult to administer, takes significant time to complete and can be difficult to interpret. However, it has characteristic response patterns for different pain syndromes such as back pain, arthritis, and cancer. The validity of this questionnaire continues to be studied. The McGill pain questionnaire consists of four different parts.

The first part consists of a human figure drawing on which you are instructed to mark the location of your pain. The second part is the pain-rating index that contains 78 words divided into 20 groups. Each set contains up to six words. Five of these groups describe tension or fear. Each word is assigned a value according to its position within a subclass.

The third part of this test asks additional questions about prior pain experiences, as well as the location of the pain and current usage of pain medications. The fourth part consists of a present pain intensity index. This aspect of the test requests a pain score from 0 to 5 with word descriptors such as no pain, mild pain, discomforting pain, distressing pain, or horrible and excruciating pain. These words also are assigned different values. All the values are added to obtain a total score. All the scores are then evaluated to attempt to assess your total pain experience.

The problem with this test is that there is no specific mechanism within the test itself to determine which component truly reflects your pain experience. The value of this test, however, is that it treats pain as a multidimensional experience. There also is a short form of the McGill pain questionnaire that has been developed. This questionnaire contains fewer words and categories than the long form. This test is sensitive to evaluations of reduction in pain experiences. This test is more useful for rapid evaluation of data following procedures or surgery.

Your psychologist may administer other tests such as the Beck Depression Inventory test. This test gives the psychologist an indication of any degree of depression that you may be experiencing. These are just two tests out of many. The purpose of these tests is to ascertain how well you are coping with your pain.

One particular psychological treatment approach that has been found to be highly effective in helping patients to reduce pain, disability and distress is Cognitive Behavioral Therapy (CBT). This type of therapy involves modifying negative thoughts related to pain and on increasing your activity level and productive functioning. This approach for pain management has been shown to be highly effective in promoting positive cognitive and behavioral changes in chronic pain patients.

Psychological treatment can be delivered individually or in a group setting. Your therapy will be tailored to your individual needs. In addition to decreasing negative thoughts, this therapy attempts to increase your activity level and productive functioning. This approach for pain management has been shown to be highly effective in promoting positive cognitive and behavioral changes in individuals with chronic pain. CBT may incorporate exercise goals set by the physical therapist, or may include recommendations made by the pain manage-ment physician for taking pain medications at prescribed time intervals.

Biofeedback is another form of beneficial therapy for pain management done by a psychologist. Biofeedback allows you to gain control over your physical processes. For example if you experience muscle pain, biofeedback can train you to relax these muscles. Biofeedback is a tool that helps sufferers alleviate their own pain. Biofeedback allows you to monitor and fine-tune the connections between your motions and health. . Biofeedback helps you recognize and control your tension and stress. Specifically, it can teach you to release the tension in your muscles and improve your circulation.

Biofeedback works by translating subtle physical changes into easy-to-read signals. A session starts when a therapist attaches sensors to your skin that measures the temperature of a finger and/or an electrode that registers the tension in your muscles. The electrodes, for instance, may be hooked up to a pair of headphones that translate tension into sound transmission. When you relax, the sound decreases but when you are tense the sound increases.

Your psychologist will help you relax, perhaps by asking you to imagine a quiet, peaceful place or by teaching you a breathing technique. As your mind becomes calm, the temperature in your finger may increase dictates that your circulation is improving. The electrodes voltage can decrease indicating that your muscles are becoming relaxed. You can become aware of your ability to influence your blood flow and relax your muscles. Biofeedback is useful for stress-related pain. Tension type headaches and migraine headaches may respond to this treatment.

In some individuals, hypnosis may help acute and chronic pain. Hypnosis has long been understood to produce varied effects in subjects. Hypnosis may be successful in pain management. Hypnosis has been shown effective in management of pain associated with childbirth, leukemia and headaches. A Viennese physician, Friederich Anton Mesmer, discovered hypnosis in the late 1700's and his technique was called Mesmerism. In England around 1843, the surgeon James Braid revisited the phenomenon of Mesmerism and renamed it hypnosis. His findings renewed interest in the subject, especially in France, where hypnosis gained popularity again as a form of pain reduction during surgery.

In the late 1800's, Bernheim and Liebeault came upon hypnosis as a treatment for physical and functional diseases. Hypnosis can help you control, diminish or redirect your pain to tolerable levels, turn pain off at your will and relax muscles, decrease stress levels and break the stress/pain cycle. In addition, hypnosis may be effective for the management pain associated with childbirth, angioplasty, phantom limb pain, leukemia, headaches and back pain. If you are to have a medical procedure and if you want hypnosis to control your pain, you must discuss this with your physician prior to committing to a hypnotist. Your physician may have a reason why hypnosis should not be used. It should be evident from reading this chapter that a psychologist trained in pain management as well as biofeedback and hypnosis can provide you with a wide variety of ways to manage your pain.

Given that no two people are alike, if you are taking any medications and begin to take nutritional supplements you should be aware that potential drug-nutrient interactions may occur and are encouraged to consult a health care professional before using any natural product. Combining certain prescription drugs and dietary supplements can lead to undesirable effects such as: diminished prescription drug effectiveness, reduced supplement effectiveness and impaired drug and/or supplement absorption.

In midlife, greater intake of omega-3 and omega-6 may be associated with lower cerebral glutamate, potentially indicating more efficient cellular reuptake of glutamate. Saturated fatty acid intake, on the other hand, was linked with poorer memory performance. These results suggest that dietary fat intake modification may be an important intervention target for the prevention of cognitive decline.[1]

Among ten studies examining foods, overall, there was a positive association between healthier foods (e.g. whole grains, fish, fruits and/or vegetables) and executive function, whereas less-healthy snack foods, sugar-sweetened beverages and red/processed meats were inversely associated with executive functioning. Taken together, evidence suggests a positive association between healthy dietary consumption and executive functioning.[2]

Nutrition performance can affect academic performance in children. A healthier diet was reported to be associated with better reading skills, but not with arithmetic skills in children.[3]

References

1.      Oleson S, Gonzales MM, Tarumi T, et al. Nutrient intake and cerebral metabolism in healthy middle-aged adults: Implications for cognitive aging. Nutr Neurosci. 2016:1-8.

2.      Cohen JF, Gorski MT, Gruber SA, Kurdziel LB, Rimm EB. The effect of healthy dietary consumption on executive cognitive functioning in children and adolescents: a systematic review. Br J Nutr. 2016;116(6):989-1000.

3.      Haapala EA, Eloranta AM, Venalainen T, et al. Diet quality and academic achievement: a prospective study among primary school children. Eur J Nutr. 2016.

# 19. PHYSICAL THERAPY

Physical therapy is an important modality that can be used to help manage your pain. Your strength and range of motion will be evaluated and treated. Your doctor will refer you to a physical therapist if he or she feels that this modality can be of some benefit to you. Physical therapists are highly trained individuals who will obtain a medical history from you and perform an examination on you.

Your physical therapist will decide which treatment is best for you based on your overall health after an evaluation. Your physical thera-pist will emphasize to you that you yourself are a major component in your rehabilitation and in the management of your chronic pain. Your physical therapist also will train you to avoid future re-injury and/or a recurrence of your pain problems.

Not only is a physical therapy evaluation a planned treatment course for your pain, you also will receive an education on future injury prevention. If you were injured in your workplace, your physical therapist will tell you how to avoid further injury in that environment. You also may be placed in a work-hardening program to enable you to become maximally conditioned for your occupation. This program duplicates your regular work duties and helps increase your muscle strength and endurance so that you can return safely back to work, hopefully without further injury.

Your physical therapist will emphasize flexibility exercises for you and show you how to do them. You have to learn to be able to move your joints without stiffness and pain. Furthermore, your physical therapist will work with you on your endurance and strength. Most importantly, your pain will be addressed. In many instances, a reduction in stiffness in combination with increases in strength and endurance will significantly reduce your pain.

Your therapist will attempt to get you back to normal daily activity as soon as possible in a safe manner. You do not want to return to activity too soon following the onset of sudden pain because you could re-injure yourself or cause yourself a worse injury. When you see your physical therapist on your first visit, you should expect the therapist to obtain a detailed medical history from you. To provide you adequate treatment, your therapist will want to know your complete medical history as well as your pain history.

The history that you tell your therapist will give the therapist important information about your pain syndrome, your prognosis, and the appropriate time that you will need to be under the physical therapist's treatments. Your therapist also will assess your behavioral response to your pain associated with your injury if you were injured in an accident or at work. If you have arthritis, your therapist will evaluate your pain input and behavior response to the arthritic pain. For example, your therapist will note if you grimace when you move your joints.

You should inform your therapist about any previous treatments that you have had for the control of your pain, including injection therapies with steroids. Your therapist may additionally want to ask questions about your social history and family history if they may be relevant to your condition. If you have back pain or neck pain, for example, a family history of rheumatoid arthritis is important for the therapist to know. If a family member has this disease, you run the risk of having this disease, which can influence what modality, you need in physical therapy.

You should not be reluctant to give your therapist your age. Many conditions occur within certain age ranges. Osteoarthritis and osteoporosis are known to occur in an older population. Your therapist must know your occupation. If your job involves heavy physical labor, for example, you may be prone to overstress of your back muscles. Tell your therapist when the pain gets worse during the day or notify your therapist if you have increased pain with certain activities. With this information, your therapist can direct an appropriate therapy program for you.

If you have had a similar pain syndrome before your most current pain syndrome, again tell your therapist. If the intensity, duration, and frequency of your pain are increasing during therapy, your therapist may want to send you back to your doctor. This is an indication that you are becoming worse with respect to what is causing your pain and not from the physical therapy.

Try to remember where your pain was when you first noticed it and keep a diary of your pain. For example, if your pain was originally in your back and then later it moved to your leg may indicate a disc rupture. If your pain has moved or spread since you first noticed it, be sure to tell your therapist. Tell the therapist what exact movements worsen your pain. Even pain with bowel movements can be an important history fact. A disc rupture can be associated with back pain during the act of defecation.

If your pain is worse in the morning and becomes progressively better during the day, this may be an indication that you have arthritis. Your therapist will need to know this information in order to prescribe the proper treatment for you. Providing a good medical history to your therapist will make it much easier for the therapist to prescribe the proper method of treatment for you.

You should write down pertinent information about yourself prior to your first physical therapy visit. Your therapist will need to know if your pain is in your bones, muscles, nerves, or all of them together. If the pain is in your bones, the pain is usually confined to that particular area. If your pain is in a nerve, the pain will usually go down your arm or leg from where the therapist is pressing on your spine or neck. If your pain is in your muscles, your physical therapist will note increased contractility of the painful muscles. Your therapist will examine the range of motion of your joints, including the range of motion of your neck and lower back.

If you have a history of dizziness or fainting, tell your therapist before you begin an exercise program. You should expect your physical therapist to look you over when you are disrobed. Your physical therapist will record how well you move and will also examine your posture. Your willingness to cooperate with your physical therapist also will be noted. Your therapist will evaluate how you walk. Your muscle size will be observed for unevenness between the right and left sides of your body from your neck down to your feet.

The color of your skin will be noted by your therapist. Sometimes if you have arthritis, there may be redness about your joints. Your hair pattern in your arms and legs will be evaluated. If you have decreased blood flow, there may be a loss of hair on your skin. Movements of your joints, neck, and lower back will be done to see how flexible you are. Any movements that are painful will be recorded and then will be addressed during your therapy session. Your therapist will decide whether heat or cold could help you with your range of motion or decrease your muscle spasms, which in turn will help decrease your pain. Your physical therapist's examination will emphasize the joints of your body as well as your muscles.

Your therapist will, furthermore, examine you for any loss of sensation in your arms and legs. For example, if you have a loss of sensation in your right shoulder, your therapist will be careful not to apply heat on this area for any significant length of time. If you have limited range of motion about your arm or leg, your therapist will work with you to increase your range of motion. A heating pad could cause a burn on your skin if you are unable to detect the sensation of heat about your shoulder. After your therapist has examined you, the therapist may call your doctor to recommend any further laboratory tests or x-rays. After the history and physical examination has been completed, your physical therapist will determine what is causing your pain problem and will design a treatment program for you based on these findings. You will be treated as a complete individual, and not as just a pain symptom. If your assessment was not done thoroughly, your treatment regimen may not help you with respect to your pain syndrome.

If you are experiencing significant pain during your therapy, immediately notify your therapist and discontinue the treatment. One goal of physical therapy is to identify the cause of your pain with an attempt to treat the cause of your pain syndrome. In addition to rehabilitating you following your injury or illness, your physical therapist will attempt to correct any mechanical flaws in your body that could lead to further injury, such as your posture.

Your therapist may do a muscle and joint stabilization program to increase your strength and flexibility. You, on the other hand, must always feel that you are a main component in your rehabilitation. If your therapist gives you exercises to do at home you follow the instructions on how to do them and do them on the prescribed schedule. Your physical therapist will treat you with exercise and strengthening techniques, but also may complement your therapy with whirlpool baths, paraffin baths, or other methods such as using electrical current.

Heat packs can provide you with surface heating, which may reduce the pain in some surface muscles in your back, arms, or legs. Ultrasound is a deep application of heat. This method can relax your deep muscles. Elastic exercise bands and medicine balls may be used to increase your arm and leg strength. The elastic bands can be used to increase your strength, and medicine balls can be used to increase your range of motion and your flexibility as well as your strength. Some physical therapists use traction for the management of your pain.

Electricity can be used to treat your pain syndrome as well. Over the years, many claims have been made for the therapeutic application of electrical current for the treatment of some pain syndromes. Electrical current is applied to your body by placement of electrodes, which are patches with adhesive that stick to your body. The current is directed over the painful areas of your body.

Electrical current can vibrate the molecules of your tissues similar to ultrasound therapy. The vibration produced by friction between the molecules of your tissues will increase your tissue temperature. As a result, heat is produced. As electrical current passes through your tissue, some nerves are excited while others are not.

It has been shown that electricity can stimulate tissue growth and repair such as bone and is sometimes used by orthopedic surgeons to stimulate bone growth following bone surgery. Sometimes stimulators can be placed following orthopedic surgery to enhance bone growth. Theoretically, the electrical current should speed up your healing time. A popular electrical current emitting device that is used frequently in pain medicine by conventional physicians, chiropractic physicians, and physical therapists is the transcutaneous electrical nerve stimulator (TENS).

A TENS unit applies electrical current to your body through electrodes that are adhered to your body. The TENS unit is used for pain control. The power source is battery operated. TENS unit therapy became popular in the late 1960s and early 1970s. The use of a TENS unit for the treatment of your chronic pain syndrome if you have neck, back, arm, and leg pain is well documented.

A TENS unit has an amplitude knob that lets your control your pain relief. These TENS units are about the size of a pager. The TENS unit patches can be placed over your muscles or nerves for the management of pain both in your muscles as well as the nerves in your arms and legs. You can use a TENS unit for the control of your pain long term without any significant side effects. Some people have allergic reactions to the adhesive in the patches.

A TENS unit can reduce your pain as well as your stress. However, you should still strive for proper body mechanics and posture. You must remember that a TENS unit is only treating your symptoms. You are in-charge of the cause of your pain. If your pain is related to poor body posture, strive to correct this problem.

Iontophoresis is another use of an electrical current to drive medications through your skin. Different medications can be applied through your skin to decrease your pain. Not only is electrical current used for pain relief, it can also speed up your tissue healing. Phonophoresis is another device that uses energy to drive medications into your body.

Traction on your neck or back can increase blood flow to the injured area of your neck or back. However, if the traction does significantly increase your pain, you must immediately notify your physical therapist. Your therapist may instruct you in stretching exercises to be done at home. You must be diligent in doing these exercises provided for you. If certain exercises that you are doing do not provide you with pain relief, ask your physical therapist to recommend some other exercises or range-of-motion methods that you can do at home or at work.

Physical therapists can help you decrease your muscle tension. Your therapist also can educate you on how to decrease muscle tension yourself. Most muscle tension is related to the stress of everyday life. While flying on an airplane for example, you may experience stress when the plane bounces around in turbulent weather. You may experience stress in your job if you have to make a presentation in front of a group. The muscles in your body naturally tense up when you are stressed.

When you experience stress, your body has a protective mechanism that increases your muscle tightness. This is an early part of the fight-or-flight response to stressful situations. This response can be helpful for your protection if you are threatened. However, when your muscles stay contracted the blood flow to your muscles decreases. This cuts off the oxygen supply to your muscles that in turn cause you to experience muscle pain.

Without oxygen, your muscles begin to hurt. Over a long time, you can develop a chronic pain syndrome as a result of your posture. Prolonged slouching over several years can make some of your muscles contract while the opposite muscles can become longer. This could cause chronic muscle pain. For example, if you slouch over a computer you can put pressure on the discs in your neck and back that act as absorbers. Slouching can cause these discs to rupture.

You should also pay attention to your neck position when you are using a telephone. If you band your neck to one side while talking on the telephone, ask your therapist if a headset could be of benefit. If you feel that your neck is stuck or "catches" in a certain position when doing exercises, that cause may be related to a small joint in your neck called a facet joint.

The bones in your neck and back stack on top of each other like blocks. Sometimes these joints can get out of position, especially if you slouch over a desk all day. Your physical therapist may be able to help you with this misalignment of your neck.

Remember if you slouch or have bad posture, your back or neck can become out of alignment. Your muscles then can pull to one side and stretch on the opposite side of your back. If you slouch over a chair for a long period of time, your spine is going to adapt to these positions. If you sit hunched over a desk all day, your ability to stand or sit upright will be compromised.

Slouching puts more pressure and stress on the discs of your back than any other posture. When you are sitting for any length of time, you should stand for 10 minutes each hour to take the pressure off the discs in your lower back. Your therapist will show you some stretching exercises to do while you are at work.

Muscles can become painful with therapy. Many athletes do physical therapy and perform resistance training and consume dietary protein as a strategy to promote anabolic adaptation. Due to its high satiety value, the regular addition of supplemented dietary protein could plausibly displace other key macronutrients such as carbohydrate in an athlete's diet. Increasing whey protein supplement dose above 20 g does not result in a measurable increase in satiety or decrease in food intake. It is important to have good nutrition habits when doing physical therapy.

Given that no two people are alike, if you are taking any medications and begin to take nutritional supplements you should be aware that potential drug-nutrient interactions may occur and are encouraged to consult a health care professional before using any natural product.

Combining certain prescription drugs and dietary supplements can lead to undesirable effects such as: diminished prescription drug effectiveness, reduced supplement effectiveness and impaired drug and/or supplement absorption.

Ginger is reported to decrease muscle pain. Four grams of ginger supplementation may be used to accelerate recovery of muscle strength following intense exercise.[1] Ginger is a popular spice used to treat a variety of maladies, including pain.

Nonsteroidal anti-inflammatory drugs (NSAIDs) are frequently used by athletes to manage and prevent pain; unfortunately, NSAIDs contribute to substantial adverse effects, including gastrointestinal (GI) dysfunction, exercise-induced bronchoconstriction, hyponatremia, impairment of connective tissue remodeling, endurance competition withdrawal, and cardiovascular disease.[2] Two grams of ginger may have anti-inflammation and analgesic effect on delayed onset muscle soreness.[3]

Reference

1.     Matsumura MD, Zavorsky GS, Smoliga JM. The Effects of Pre-Exercise Ginger Supplementation on Muscle Damage and Delayed Onset Muscle Soreness. Phytother Res. 2015;29(6):887-893.

2.     Wilson PB. Ginger (Zingiber officinale) as an Analgesic and Ergogenic Aid in Sport: A Systemic Review. J Strength Cond Res. 2015;29(10):2980-2995.

3.     Hoseinzadeh K, Daryanoosh F, Baghdasar PJ, Alizadeh H. Acute effects of ginger extract on biochemical and functional symptoms of delayed onset muscle soreness. Med J Islam Repub Iran. 2015;29:261.

The pathology that affects your lower back also affects your neck. In other words, muscles, nerves, ligaments, discs and facet joints may cause neck pain. At any given time, neck pain affects 10 percent of the general population in the United States. Neck pain is a frequent reason why patients seek medical attention. Neck pain can range from mild discomfort to severe and throbbing and is experienced by everyone at some point in his or her life.

Neck pain is caused by conditions that compress nerves or irritate the outer part of discs that are cushions between the bones in your neck. Ligaments in the front and in the back of your bones in your neck can cause pain because they have many pain fibers within these ligaments. These ligaments are called the anterior and posterior longitudinal ligaments.

The vertebrae in your neck stack on top of each other and are separated by discs. They form joints called facet joints where each vertebra joint. The outer capsule of each joint has a rich supply of pain fibers. The outer capsule holds the top and bottom of the facet joint together not unlike a clamshell. If this capsule is pulled or stretched by an injury, the joint can become loose and make the joint unstable. This instability can cause neck pain.

If your neck becomes misaligned, you can also develop significant neck pain. Over time, the bones and joints in your neck can wear out as well. This is called degenerative disc or joint disease or in medical terms is called osteoarthritis. The disc between your bones can rupture. Your facet joints in your neck can deteriorate and cause you to develop chronic neck pain. Your neck muscles can become tense as well and cause you additional neck pain.

Neck pain in general does not occur as often as low back pain. There-fore, the overall cost of neck pain to society is much less than that of lower back pain. There is fewer work days lost and less medications prescribed in patients with neck pain when compared to lower back pain. Your head weighs between 10 and 12 pounds. The bones in your neck are relatively small in comparison to your head. Your neck muscles are necessary to hold your head in a proper position. Your neck muscles must be strong to hold your head up. Try holding a bowling ball vertically for as long as you can. You will notice that your arm muscles get tired easily. The same analogy is true with respect to your neck muscles tiring from holding your head up.

The bones in your neck that are called vertebral bodies contain many pain fibers. If you fracture one of the bones in your neck, you can have severe pain. The tissue wrapper (periosteum) around your neck vertebra can be injured. The fracture of a bone in your neck can cause abnormal stress to the ligaments, muscles, and joints around the fracture as well as injury to your periosteum (an outer wrapper around the vertebral body).

Osteoporosis is a weakening of your bones from a loss of your bone density and calcium. This disease can cause small, tiny fractures in the bones of your neck and in turn can be a cause of your pain. Osteoporosis can be a source of severe neck pain.

Discs are cushions between the bones in your neck. These discs act as shock absorbers in between your bones. The cushions are important because without them your neck bones would stack on top of each other. Remember the periosteum and the pain fibers contained in the periosteum. Without these cushions, you would have terrible neck pain.

In the very center of your disc in your neck is a thick fluid like substance called a nucleus pulposus. This fluid ball is surrounded by an outer tough fiber called an annulus. Annulus is Latin for "outer ring." When the annulus bulges, pain fibers on the outer aspect of this structure can cause pain signals to be propagated. A fluid nucleus pulposus acts as a ball bearing that enables you to bend your head forward and backward or from side to side. It also is a ball bearing when you rotate your neck.

The ligaments around your disc prevent your neck from having excessive motion. Otherwise, your bones would sit on a fluid-filled ball and flop around like a Slinky toy. You can imagine that your neck would not be very stable without ligaments. Your annulus at its outer layer has many pain fibers. Neck degeneration flattens your discs. When the disc looses height, it pushes your annulus outward. This action stimulates pain fiber activity. This is why you hurt constantly as your disc degenerate.

Magnetic resonance imaging (MRI) and computerized tomography scanning (CT) can help your doctor identify any bone or disc abnormalities that may be a source of your neck pain. Be aware, however, that an abnormal imaging study does not necessarily mean that you will have neck pain. It is possible that you can have a ruptured disc in your neck and you may not experience any neck pain.

There is a normal C-shaped curve in your neck . Your neck bones form a C curve with the C part of the curve located in the middle of your neck. The C curve is called a lordosis. The curve is sharper at the lower level of your neck. The curve in your neck determines your posture. If you have a neck injury, the muscles in your neck may pull your neck in a straight line and the curve is obliterated. If you have an X-ray following an injury, your doctor may note that your neck is straight as opposed to being curved. If your neck muscles are in spasm your neck may be straight.

A whiplash injury which will be described in this chapter can cause your neck muscles to develop spasm. This will cause your neck to straighten. If you look at your X ray, you will not see your normal C curve in your neck. Normally your neck is not straight. It should have a curve. Remember that the muscles of your neck stabilize your neck. Following an injury, your neck muscles may be stretched and com-pressed.

Trauma can cause your neck muscles to contract without relaxing which is called a muscle spasm. Muscle spasms compress the arteries that bring oxygen to your neck muscles and nerves. If your blood flow is decreased, acid (lactic acid is formed in your muscle tissue). Tissue oxygen deprivation causes pain.

This is similar to heart pain when you have a heart attack. Muscle relaxant medications, massage therapy or injections into your neck muscles can relax your muscles and restore blood flow. This will decrease your pain. The outer ring of your disc, called the annulus, will contain the nucleus pulposus within its structure. Think of this anatomy as a jelly doughnut. The jelly in the doughnut is held in place by the outer doughnut ring.

A whiplash injury can be extremely painful. To understand the concept of a whiplash injury, consider that your head is as if it is a bowling ball attached to a flexible whip called your neck. At the time of an accident, your bowling ball flies away from the traumatic event but fortunately or unfortunately, it is still connected to your neck. This connection causes your neck and head to snap like a whip that can cause an injury not only to your neck but also to your brain.

Whiplash is a relatively common injury that occurs to a patient's neck following a sudden acceleration–deceleration force, most commonly from motor vehicle accidents. Whiplash is the common name for neck sprains. Whiplash associated disorders describe a more severe and chronic condition. It was known for many years that accidents involving rear-end collisions caused more neck pain than side-impact or frontal-impact collisions. The cervical spine is subjected to a compressive force from weight of the head during a rear-impact collision. The problem occurs when the body starts to move forward and the head remains. Subsequently, the head begins its movement backward and the weight of the head compresses down on the cervical spine.

The exact injury mechanism that causes whiplash injuries is unknown but may be caused by stretching the anterior longitudinal ligament. While cervical myofascial injury is the most common problem with whiplash-associated disorders, the cervical facet joints are routinely injured in these accidents. Whiplash-associated disorders may result from rear end or side-impact motor vehicle collisions, but can also occur during diving and other accidents. Symptoms of this disorder include neck pain, neck swelling, tenderness along the back of your neck, muscle spasms, difficulty moving your neck and headaches.

Whiplash-associated disorders predispose one to premature degenerative changes. A history of psychiatric disease was more common in patients with chronic symptoms. The dominating psychiatric diagnosis both before and after the accident was depression. Psychiatric morbidity may be a patient-related risk factor for chronic pain symptoms after a whiplash injury.

Four grades of Whiplash-Associated Disorder have been defined by the Quebec Task Force on whiplash-associated disorders: Grade 1: complaints of neck pain, stiffness or tenderness only but no physical signs are noted by the examining physician, Grade 2: neck complaints and the examining physician finds decreased range of motion and point tenderness in the neck, Grade 3: decreased range of motion plus neurological signs such as decreased deep tendon reflexes, weakness, insomnia and sensory deficits and Grade 4: neck complaints and fracture or dislocation, or injury to the spinal cord.

Most whiplash injuries resolve with conservative treatment. Chiropractic and/or physical therapy are very effective modalities. If these modalities fail, trigger point injections or facet joint injections may be of benefit. A facet rhizotomy may be done if the pain persists. If none of these modalities resolve the pain, a consultation with a surgeon is indicated.

You are probably aware that if you sustained an injury to your head and if your neck bends to far toward one of the sides of your body, the holes (called foramina) for the nerves going to your arms on the side where the head bends will be narrowed. This can cause you to have a nerve injury because the closed hole can compress one of your nerves coming off of your spinal cord. On the opposite side, the holes where the nerves emerge from your spinal cord will be opened.

When your head is thrown to the side, as frequently happens when you suffer a whiplash injury, the side on which the head is thrown to can compress the facet joints on that side of your neck. On the opposite side the facet joints are opened. Either of these maneuvers can cause you to have a facet joint injury or can cause you to suffer significant pain.

If you have arthritis, osteophytes can irritate or compress one or more of your nerves. Osteophytes are abnormal bone growths. Osteophytes themselves are not painful. However, when they brush over your nerves or ligaments, they can cause you to have neck pain. Osteophytes, if they occur, are usually pointed. If one of your nerves brushes up against one of these osteophytes, or if the osteophytes compress your or irritate one of your nerves which can cause you to experience mild to moderate pain.

Steroid injections in and around your nerves can decrease the swelling of the nerve and decrease your pain. Sometimes your doctor may give you steroids by mouth. The problem with oral steroids is that they can cause you to have a significant weight gain. The injection places a tiny amount of steroids at the area of your pain.

Oral steroids have to go to your stomach and pass out of your gastroinetstinal system to reach your bloodstream. The total amount of the steroid that will reach your swollen nerves will vary. This is why pain medicine doctors advocate the use of special needles to place steroids at the level of your nerve swelling. The amount of drug placed at your nerve is more reliable than that given by mouth.

The muscles in the base of your skull can compress a nerve that comes off of your spinal cord and travels to the top of your head. This is called the occipital nerve (figure 2). If a tight muscle compresses this nerve, you can develop a headache called an occipital headache. If you put some heat over the muscle that is compressing this nerve, it can relax the muscle and relieve your headache. Occipital headaches can be treated by a neurologist. Sometimes an injection of a steroid at the occipital nerve can decrease your headache. An epidural steroid injection may also be helpful. Cryoanalgesia (freezing your nerve) may also be of benefit. Botulism toxin (Botox) may also be of benefit as well.

The picture of the model looks at your neck from a posterior (rear) view. In addition to similar structures in your low back, you also have a spinal cord that can be a source of pain. A syringomyelia or defect in your spinal cord can be a source of your neck pain. A syringomyelia is an abnormal fluid space within the spinal cord that is sometimes associated with a tumor or trauma of the spinal cord, or a Chiari malformation. If the abnormal fluid channel or "syrinx" enlarges enough, it can cause pressure on the nearby nerve fibers in the spinal cord resulting in numbness in the arms and or legs. In such cases, consideration can be given to operating on the syrinx in order to drain it.

Nerves that come off your spinal cord travel to the top of your head. Some of these nerves form the Greater and Lesser Occipital Nerves. If these nerves are compressed from trauma, muscle spasm or degenerative disc disease or facet joint degeneration, you may develop pain that begins in the base of your skull and then travels to the top of your skull. The treatment of this pain consists of anticonvulsant drugs, anti-depressant drugs or injections with steroids and local anesthetics. The nerves can be deadened by freezing them (cryoanalgesia) or with phenol. If the pain persists, a peripheral nerve stimulator can be implanted that may decrease your pain.

If you do develop degenerative disc disease in your neck, you will have decreased range of motion about your neck. The decreased range of motion around your neck is an early indication that you are developing degeneration of the discs and joints in your neck. You will have trouble turning your head and attempting to look behind you. Looking up or down also can be difficult as well as painful.

If you have a severe state of contractions of a muscle in your neck, you may have severe pain. This prolonged contraction of a neck muscle is called torticollis. This usually occurs on one side of your neck. Your head is usually twisted to one side with your chin pointing to the opposite side. Torticollis usually results from disease or an injury to your brain or spinal cord. Injuries to the muscles of your neck can also be a cause of torticollis as well. Sometimes an injection of botulism can relieve your pain.

Some people also pass out when their head is bent backward because of compression of arteries that go to their brain. It is important to let your doctor know if you have experienced any of these problems after going to a hair salon. If you have significant pathology you should avoid hyper extending your neck. You should be aware of your posture. You should use a telephone headset if you have a job that requires considerable telephone time. Avoidance of improper neck posture while using a telephone can contribute to your neck pain. You should avoid the use of large pillows. A flat pillow can keep your neck in a proper position while you sleep.

Given that no two people are alike, if you are taking any medications and begin to take nutritional supplements you should be aware that potential drug-nutrient interactions may occur and are encouraged to consult a health care professional before using any natural product. Combining certain prescription drugs and dietary supplements can lead to undesirable effects such as: diminished prescription drug effectiveness, reduced supplement effectiveness and impaired drug and/or supplement absorption.

Potential causes of the age-related degeneration of intervertebral discs include declining nutrition, loss of viable cells, cell senescence, post-translational modification of matrix proteins, accumulation of degraded matrix molecules, and fatigue failure of the matrix. The most important of these mechanisms appears to be decreasing nutrition of the central disc that allows accumulation of cell waste products and degraded matrix molecules, impairs cell nutrition, and causes a fall in pH levels that further compromises cell function and may cause cell death.[1]

A program has been developed for chronic pain sufferers, primarily those with low back and cervical spine pain. The treatment is a six-week interdisciplinary program including relaxation training, gradually increasing exercise, and significant education on behavioral and exercise strategies and nutrition for long-term pain management. This program is inexpensive, cost efficient, and may be implemented easily in a variety of settings.[2]

Omega-3 fatty acids appear just as effective as NSAIDs, if not more so, in relieving certain kinds of neck and back pain.

References

1.      Buckwalter JA. Aging and degeneration of the human inter-vertebral disc. Spine (Phila Pa 1976). 1995;20(11):1307-1314.

2.      Wells MJ, Peay A. Interdisciplinary Treatment of Musculo-skeletal Pain: The EMPOWER Program. J Back Musculoskelet Rehabil. 1993;3(1):54-63.

# 21. BACK PAIN

Low back pain has many causes; injury, stress, poor posture, or aging. Many people experience back pain, and there are various treatment methods available. In some instances utilizing proper posture techniques and performing stretching exercises during the day can prevent back pain. Your back consists of a large number of bones called vertebrae that are separated from one another by cushions called discs. These discs act as shock absorbers between each bone in your spine.

The bones stack on top of each other like blocks and form joints called facet joints. The purpose of your spinal skeleton is protects your spinal cord from injury. There are foramina, which are holes in each vertebra. The nerves off of your spinal cord go through these holes and go to your arms, legs, and organs within your body.

Your spine is kept in place by muscles in your back that maintain your posture. Your muscles also make your back stable during movement. You have many muscles in your back. Any one of these muscles can cause you to have lower back pain. In addition to muscles, you have ligaments that attach each bone in your spine to both the one above and the one below. Ligaments also are necessary to give your back stability. Your ligaments contain pain fibers and can be a source of your back pain as well.

Most of your lower back pain is usually mechanical in nature. This means that there is usually an abnormal alignment of your bones and/or joints that can cause you to have back pain. Figure 1 demonstrates the anatomy of your lumbar spine. You should note that the discs separate the vertebral bodies. The discs in this model are of a normal size. The nerves come out of foramina and ultimately go down your leg. The foramina are normal in appearance.

When your back degenerates, all or part of your back anatomy changes. These changes may cause you to experience pain. Disc degeneration however, does not mean that you will experience pain. Patients with degenerative disc disease in many instances do not experience pain. Degenerative disc disease is a normal aging process. This process may be accelerated by smoking cigarettes. You should note that the discs separate the vertebral bodies. The discs in the model (Figure 1) are of a normal size. The nerves come out of foramina and ultimately go down your leg. The foramina are normal in appearance.

When the discs degenerate, they lose water (desiccate). As a result, your disc height becomes smaller. Your overall height becomes less as well. The loss of disc height places stress on your facet joints which may cause you to experience facet joint pain. The foramina can become smaller as well which can cause pressure on one or more of your nerve roots. This may cause you to experience pain down your leg which is called sciatica.

You have five bones in your lower back that are called lumbar vertebrae. Your spine functions to support you when you are standing, walking, bending, pushing, and pulling. Your back must perform repetitive tasks on a daily basis without failure. Most of your everyday back pains are not serious. Your back pain is most probably related to a muscle strain or a ligament sprain from doing an activity that you are not used to doing. You should however, never ignore your back pain. You should be concerned if your back pain goes down your legs. If your back pain is associated with weakness of your legs or numbness or difficulty walking, you need to see a doctor.

If you have damage to your spinal cord, you may become paralyzed. If this happens, you may lose all control of your bowel and bladder. Back pain is the most common cause of disability for workers younger than age 45. Back pain is responsible for 15 percent of work absenteeism in developed countries. Approximately 5 percent of the work force is disabled by back pain yearly. Attempts to prevent back pain have not been proven to be effective. In 1990 in the United States, there were 15 million office visits to doctors for lower back pain. This accounts for approximately 3 percent of all visits to doctors. The number of visits to chiropractors was even greater.

The rates for surgery in the United States have increased over the past 20 years. The rate of surgery for back pain in the United States is greater than in most other countries. Following the onset of back pain, there can be a recurrence of lower back pain in a person within 1 year and a 75 percent recurrence in a person's lifetime. Sixty-five percent of patients usually recover from an episode of back pain within six weeks. At 12 weeks, 85 percent of those with back pain are essentially pain free. If you have pain for more than 12 weeks, it is unlikely that you will receive significant relief of your back pain.

If you have been off of work for more than 26 weeks because of back pain, you will probably not be able to return back to work. If you receive compensation from a workmen's compensation insurance carrier or compensation following a motor vehicle accident, your chances of returning to work are significantly decreased. If you are over 50 years of age, you can expect to have problems with your back and also have limitations in your activity due to back pain. Back pain from heavy physical work is common by age 50. Back pain is an unavoidable part of your life.

If you do a job that requires physical labor, you can expect to have back pain when you are 50 years of age or older. Even people who have not done heavy physical work can begin experiencing increased back pain by age 50. You should realize that it would be difficult to decrease your back pain if you have become inactive. For this reason, you should do aerobic exercise to prevent back pain. You also can use exercise to treat back pain. The muscles in your back must be strong in order to support your back. This is the reason that you must do regular exercise activity.

You may have a job where you must do repetitive lifting or twisting. This can injure your back as well as place wear and tear on your discs. If you have a job where you sit all day at a computer desk or at a workbench and you slouch, your back can become misaligned. You may have suffered sports injuries to your back. If you enjoy gardening, you can cause yourself to have back pain if you are doing a considerable amount of digging or lifting.

If your back is not conditioned and strong, try to avoid heavy lifting and strenuous recreational activities. As you grow older, your discs lose their elastic properties and they become thinner and can become wafer thin. As the discs in your back decrease in height, your overall height decreases. As your discs begin to shrink, pressure from the bones above and below can cause your discs to press outward. This is called a disc bulge.

Sometimes a disc bulge can press on one of your nerves. A disc bulge is not a disc rupture. However, a disc bulge can press on one of your nerves coming off of your spinal cord and can cause you significant pain. If your pain persists and you develop numbness, you may ultimately have to have surgery to remove a portion of this bulge off of your nerve.

In the very center of your disc is a thick liquid. Liquids cannot be compressed. If you bend a certain way or attempt to lift a heavy object in an awkward position, the fluid inside of your disc can burst through the outer ring of your disc. This is called a disc herniation or disc rupture and can cause you to experience significant pain.

The liquid material that bursts outside of your disc is highly acidic. This acidic liquid can cause your nerves, your ligaments and your muscles to become swollen and inflamed and you can develop severe pain. Most of the origins of your back pain discussed are mechanical in nature. However, injuries to your discs between your backbones can cause you to have pain. Remember that your discs are also made up of cartilage as well.

It is important for you to understand that a herniated disc does not mean that you will have back pain. In fact 37 % of individuals in the United

States have disc herniations but never experience any back pain. A disc herniation furthermore, does not mean that you are disabled or will become disabled. A disc herniation does not mean that you will need surgery. Most disc herniations are treated conservatively with medications, physical therapy, chiropractic therapy or epidural steroid injections. If you do require surgery, you should not expect to be disabled after surgery. In most instances you will be able to return to work unless you have to do extremely heavy lifting. Most professional athletes return back to work following disc surgery.

The surgery rate in the United States has increased over the past 20 years. The rate of surgery for back pain in the United States is greater than in most other countries. Following the onset of back pain, there can be a recurrence of lower back pain in a person within 1 year and a 75 percent recurrence in a person's lifetime. Sixty-five percent of patients usually recover from an episode of back pain within six weeks. At 12 weeks, 85 percent of those with back pain are essentially pain free.

If you have pain for more than 12 weeks, it is unlikely that you will receive significant relief of your back pain. If you have been off of work for more than 26 weeks because of back pain, you will probably not be able to return back to work. If you receive compensation from a workmen's compensation insurance carrier or compensation following a motor vehicle accident, your chances of returning to work are significantly decreased. If you are over 50 years of age, you can expect to have problems with your back and also have limitations in your activity due to back pain. Back pain from heavy physical work is common by age 50. Back pain is an unavoidable part of your life.

If you do a job that requires physical labor, you can expect to have back pain when you are 50 years of age or older. Even people who have not done heavy physical work can begin experiencing increased back pain by age 50. You should realize that it would be difficult to decrease your back pain if you have become inactive. For this reason, you should do aerobic exercise to prevent back pain. You also can use exercise to treat back pain. The muscles in your back must be strong in order to support your back. This is the reason that you must do regular exercise activity..

You may have a job where you must do repetitive lifting or twisting. This can injure your back as well as place wear and tear on your discs. If you have a job where you sit all day at a computer desk or at a workbench and you slouch, your back can become misaligned. You may have suffered sports injuries to your back. If you enjoy gardening, you can cause yourself to have back pain if you are doing a considera-ble amount of digging or lifting.

In some situations, activity does not cause back pain.  If you sleep on a soft mattress, you may awaken with significant spine pain.  A soft mattress will cause your back to become out of alignment.  Chiroprac-tic therapy may be necessary to realign your back which should relieve your back pain.

If you develop spinal stenosis (narrowing of the bones of your spine that choke your nerves that run vertical or foraminal stenosis that occurs when the openings for your nerves to your legs become narrow.  Activity does not cause this condition, but activity can cause you to experience pain.  You have to walk bent over.  You will have pain in your calves.  Sitting will relieve your pain.  This is called neuroclaudication

Figure 1.Disc herniation.

Your discs and cartilage are elastic and functions as a cushion be-tween your backbones. These discs absorb the impact of your body motion. If your discs put pressure on the nerves going to your leg, your leg may become numb or you could develop a foot drop. You must seek medical attention if this happens. When your doctor examines you, you may have no reflexes in your leg on the side of your pain.

When you reach age 50, the liquid center of your discs, called the nu-cleus pulposus, becomes dry and less elastic. Pressure on your discs can cause them to protrude and cause your discs to keep protruding until they may become compressed around one of the nerves going to your legs. When this happens, it can compress your nerve. If your leg becomes numb and weak, you will probably become a candidate for surgery. You will need consultation with a neurosurgeon or an orthopedic surgeon.

Aging also can cause your facet joints to become calcified and the surfaces of your joints can become irregular. Excessive wear and tear over time may make your facet joints become misaligned. If your facet joints become misaligned, one of the joint components can move forward and can again compress one of the nerves going to your legs causing pain and possibly numbness and weakness. A normal spine that has been maintained with exercise, proper posture, and range-of-motion exercises enables you to bend and rotate your back without pain. These exercises will help you maintain adequate range of motion for your back. These movements also can help increase blood flow to your discs.

Increased blood flow can encourage your discs to heal and can even prevent scar tissue from forming around your nerves that were temporarily injured. In some instances, you may need to seek chiropractic therapy to realign your back. If the bones in your back are properly aligned, your nerves should be able to transmit normal impulses to your muscles to allow your muscles to function in an optimal fashion.

If there is some entrapment of your nerves by pressure from adjacent body structures, your nervous system cannot function properly. If you are overweight and do not exercise and do not use proper posture, your back muscles and discs will become progressively weaker. Your discs can decrease is size. This occurrence is referred to as degenerative disc disease (figure 3). This is not a disease but normal aging. You will then be prone to a disc rupture if you perform a strenuous activity. This is the reason why you need to maintain a healthful lifestyle that includes exercise.

Cigarette smoking can cause your discs to degenerate. This may be a reason why cigarette smokers have a higher incidence of back pain. Cessation of smoking will not allow your discs to regenerate however. Nicotine can also interfere with the absorption of pain medicines into your blood stream from your stomach and your small intestine. Many smokers who stopped smoking have noticed that their pain medications became more effective. You should also be aware that if you are a smoker and need back surgery, you might not heal properly.

Many surgeons will make you stop smoking at least 4 weeks before doing back surgery. Your discs and cartilage are elastic and functions as a cushion between your backbones. These discs absorb the impact of your body motion. If your discs put pressure on the nerves going to your leg, your leg may become numb or you could develop a foot drop. You must seek medical attention if this happens. When your doctor examines you, you may have no reflexes in your leg on the side of your pain.

When you reach age 50, the liquid center of your discs, called the nucleus pulposus, becomes dry and less elastic. Pressure on your discs can cause them to protrude and cause your discs to keep protruding until they may become compressed around one of the nerves going to your legs. When this happens, it can compress your nerve. If your leg becomes numb and weak, you will probably become a candidate for surgery. You will need consultation with a neurosurgeon or an orthopedic surgeon.

Aging also can cause your facet joints to become calcified and the surfaces of your joints can become irregular. Excessive wear and tear over time may make your facet joints become misaligned. If your facet joints become misaligned, one of the joint components can move forward and can again compress one of the nerves going to your legs causing pain and possibly numbness and weakness.

A normal spine that has been maintained with exercise, proper posture, and range-of-motion exercises enables you to bend and rotate your back without pain. These exercises will help you maintain adequate range of motion for your back. These movements also can help increase blood flow to your discs.

Increased blood flow can encourage your discs to heal and can even prevent scar tissue from forming around your nerves that were tempo-rarily injured. In some instances, you may need to seek chiropractic therapy to realign your back. If the bones in your back are properly aligned, your nerves should be able to transmit normal impulses to your muscles to allow your muscles to function in an optimal fashion.

If there is some entrapment of your nerves by pressure from adjacent body structures, your nervous system cannot function properly. If you are overweight and do not exercise and do not use proper posture, your back muscles and discs will become progressively weaker.

Your discs can decrease is size. This occurrence is referred to as de-generative disc disease. This is not a disease but normal aging. You will then be prone to a disc rupture if you perform a strenuous activity. This is the reason why you need to maintain a healthful lifestyle that includes exercise.

In degenerative disc disease, your discs decrease in height and the ends of your bones become irregular. The disc spaces are where the discs are located between the bones.

Every patient who has low back pain does not need a MRI or CT scan. A plain X ray is cheaper and provides significant information about your back. In figure 3, the spaces between the discs are somewhat narrow. Osteophytes are present on the vertebral bodies. This X ray indicates that some wear and tear of your back is occurring.

Preventative pain medicine is just as important as the treatment of many pain problems. Where your backbone and pelvis meet, they form a joint called the sacroiliac joint (figure 4). Your sacroiliac joint can be a source of your back pain as well. This joint has a thick capsule that has strong ligaments both in the front and the back of your joint. Other ligaments also help to form and support this joint. The joint is C shaped.

As you become older, the cartilage that attaches to your pelvic bone degenerates faster than the cartilage in your sacrum. As a result this joint which is called the sacroiliac joint can become unstable. It can be a cause of your pain as well. Related to hormone changes that occur during pregnancy, the ligament becomes loose. This is the reason that many pregnant women experience pain in their sacroiliac joints that can last after the birth of their baby until the ligament becomes stronger. Sometimes the pain from your sacroiliac joint can cause pain to go down your leg. In other instances the pain will be referred to your hip or may just be present in your sacroiliac joint. The gluteal muscle over this joint may hurt as well.

You may notice pain in your back when you roll over in bed or when you get out of a car. Furthermore, you can have pain when you go up or down steps. If the muscle over your sacroiliac joint is tight, it can cause you to have pain. A bone scan is helpful in diagnosing sacroiliac arthritis.

During this procedure, a very small dose of a radioactive dye is injected into your veins. After the radioactive dye has had time to go to your joints, pictures are taken with a camera of your sacroiliac joint. If you have arthritis, there will be darkened areas in your joints that will show up on the scan. Usually plain x-rays are not sufficient to diagnose problems with your sacroiliac joint. The treatment of this problem consists of physical therapy.

A type of Velcro belt called an SI belt can be used to hold your joint in place. Stabilization of your joint can decrease your pain. If you have no relief from these methods, your pain-medicine doctor can inject a steroid and local anesthetic into your joint under X-ray needle guidance. These methods should rid you of your pain. If your pain does persist, destruction of the nerves that goes to your joint can be done with either heat or cold. This is called a rhizotomy.

Occasionally, a surgeon may have to stabilize your joint surgically. Nonsteroidal anti-inflammatory medications also can be very helpful for the management of pain in your sacroiliac joint. Because the pain involves a joint, muscle relaxants may not be of any benefit.

If you have a disc herniation, a CAT scan or an MRI can diagnose your pathology. Your lower back is made up of five bones called lumbar vertebrae. The lower part of your back below these bones is called the sacrum. It is made up of five fused bones. Your pelvis anchors here. Your tailbone is called a coccyx.

If you sit in a chair correctly or in the seat of your car correctly, you are keeping all of these bones properly aligned. Each bone then bears the full weight of the bone above it. It is reported that proper alignment of your back can help build bone mass. This is important if anyone in your family has a history of osteoporosis.

Discography is a way of diagnosing whether or not that you have disc-related pain. An MRI and CT scan can show a disc herniation. However, these imaging studies cannot define pain. A discogram is an injec-tion of material into your disc. The pressure in your disc is then measured. You should have a relatively high pressure when material is injected into the center of your disc. If your disc leaks, the leakage of the acidic nucleus pulposus can cause you to have pain.

When your nucleus pulposus leaks out of your disc it hardens just like glue out of its tube. Sciatica is a pain that is felt in your back and the outer side of your thigh, leg, and foot. It is usually caused by degeneration of one of the discs between your backbones. When the disc protrudes laterally off to the side, it can compress the nerves in your lower back. Usually the last two or three nerves are compressed on the side of your pain. The onset of sciatica can be sudden. Furthermore, it can be brought on if you are performing an awkward lifting position or if you are doing a twisting movement such as raking the leaves.

Patients who have sciatica usually have stiff backs and have pain when they attempt any movement. You may have numbness in your leg as well as weakness associated with your sciatica. Bed rest for 24 hours may decrease your pain. If you have significant weakness and pain, nonsteroidal anti-inflammatory medication can help. If this medication does not provide you with relief, your pain-medicine doctor may want to inject the sciatic nerve with some numbing medicine and a steroid.

If you still have pain after conservative treatments have been tried, a surgeon may need to do a surgical procedure to get either a muscle or disc off your nerve to relieve your pain. In addition to degenerative changes in the back and joints as being common causes of back pain, the most common cause of back pain is muscle tension in the lower back. Approximately 80 percent of people living in the United States will experience one incident of an aching back at some time in their lives.

Be aware that stress can play a major role in the origin of your lower back pain. If you are frightened or nervous, your muscles become tense. When your muscles tighten, the tightness of the muscle can progress to muscle spasms where the muscles contract and pull.

You should know that the muscles in your back are not under your control when they become tense. Misalignment of your back due to poor posture or other mechanical strains such as slouching in a chair can cause you to have back pain. If you sit over a computer desk with your back rounded, your muscles are going to adapt to that position. Often the muscle fiber length will change to conform to your improper position. When this happens, your spine is going to adapt to these positions as well.

You must remember that hunching over a desk or slouching in a chair can press some muscles and elongate other muscles. Also, tendons, joints, and ligaments that support your back are affected. Some of the ligaments are stretched while some are compressed. When you slouch or when you sit rounded over, you can compress some of the facet joints while opening other facet joints. You must remember that your lower back supports your body.

Your lower body extends from your ribcage to your pelvis. Not only does your lower back include muscles of your lower back, it also includes muscles around your stomach. Muscles in your back, includ-ng the muscles around your stomach, attach the front of the spine to the hips. At the attachment of the hips, the muscles are anchored. Persistent slouching will eventually affect your posture. When your posture causes your back to be misaligned, you will develop pain.

As previously mentioned, the discs in between the bones in your back can be a source of back pain. Again, you must be aware that slouching puts more excessive pressure and stress on your discs than does any other posture. Slouching can, therefore, decrease the blood flow to your discs and cause your discs to lose their height and begin to calcify, which is called degeneration. This condition can cause you chronic pain.

You can have chronic pain following back surgery. This is usually a result of how your body heals and is not something caused by your surgeon. Scar can form around your nerves that go from your back to your hips and legs. This is called a failed back syndrome. Repeat surgery is usually ineffective. If medications do not provide you with sufficient pain relief, you may need a dorsal column stimulator that is discussed elsewhere in this book.

Slouching in a chair and at a desk also can cause you to have chronic pain by compressing the nerves that come off of your spinal cord and go toyour legs. Your lower back has a natural C curve at the lower end of your back. This normal curve is called a lordodic curve.

Chronic slouching can straighten this normal C curve in your back. This misalignment will affect your discs, muscles, ligaments, and joints. Look at your posture in your mirror. If your posture is abnormal, you must correct it. If you cannot do it yourself, you may want to visit a chiropractor or physical therapist to help you with this problem.

Be aware that as you age one of the first consequences of aging is unfortunately in your discs. Before your hair turns gray or before you lose hair and develop wrinkles, changes usually occur in one of both of the two lower discs in your back. The lower discs in your lumbar spine essentially do not have a blood supply from arteries to your disc after age 12. The blood supply of your discs must come from the ends of your vertebral bodies. Most of the oxygen and sugar that goes to your discs comes from the ends of your vertebral bodies. Your discs need these nutrients. If you smoke, you decrease these important nutrients to your disc that accelerates the degeneration of your discs.

After your discs have begun to age, the joints around your vertebral bodies will degenerate. Remember that your bones stack up on top of each other and that the back of your bones forms joints with the bones above and below your discs called facet joints. As your disc narrows as a result of degeneration, the space between your discs narrows. Not only do you decrease your height, you also compress your facet joints.

Disc compression causes your discs to wear out faster. The facet joints in your spine work to stabilize your spine. As your joints deteriorate, you will lose motion as your age increases. Spondylolisthesis can be another cause of your back pain. This occurs when one of your bones slips upon the one below it. This is usually hereditary in origin.

Trauma can also cause this disorder. However, when one bone slips over the other, it can cause pain in your facet joints and sometimes it can compress the nerves coming off of your spinal cord going to your legs. Vertebral body slippage can put stress on your ligaments that can cause pain as well. Usually surgery is not needed for minor slippage. Your pain can be frequently controlled with NSAIDs. Occasionally a steroid injection into your epidural space or a steroid into your facet joint can help you control your pain. Sometimes chiropractic therapy can help you in the management of your pain if you have this syndrome.

There are many causes of low back pain. Fortunately, most low back pain can be managed with conservative treatment. Preventive care is extremely important. You should be aware of your posture. You should exercise. If you smoke, you should begin a smoking cessation program. A walking program can strengthen your back. You should have a firm mattress.

Alignment of your spine may need to be done on occasion. If your muscles become tight, you should do relaxation exercises. Biofeedback can help relax your back muscles. If you are going to lift a heavy object, you should keep your back straight and bend your knees.

Given that no two people are alike, if you are taking any medications and begin to take nutritional supplements you should be aware that potential drug-nutrient interactions may occur and are encouraged to consult a health care professional before using any natural product. Combining certain prescription drugs and dietary supplements can lead to undesirable effects such as: diminished prescription drug effectiveness, reduced supplement effectiveness and impaired drug and/or supplement absorption.

Back pain brings about one of the heaviest burden of disease. Despite much research, this condition remains poorly understood, and effective treatments are frustratingly elusive. Thus, researchers in the field need to consider new hypotheses. Vitamin C (ascorbic acid) is an essential cofactor for collagen crosslinks, a key determinant of ligament, tendon, and bone quality. Recent studies have reported high frequency of hypovitaminosis C in the general population. We hypothesized that lack of vitamin C contributes to poor collagen properties and back pain.[1]

Exercise and nutrition to help treat these potential underlying and contributory mechanisms of spine pathology.[2]

A study was conducted to examine the association between Modic classification and the eating habits in patients with degenerative disc disease (DDD) and to determine the influence of nutrition on disease severity. The frequency with which patients with low back pain consumed water, salt, fast food, eggs, milk, yogurt, cheese, whole wheat bread, white bread, butter, and margarine was studied and recorded. Modic changes on MRI imaging which indicates the severity of DDD, seem to be correlated to patients' dietary habits. Patients with healthy eating habits had less lumbar disc pathology.[3]

References

1.      Dionne CE, Laurin D, Desrosiers T, et al. Serum vitamin C and spinal pain: a nationwide study. Pain. 2016;157(11):2527-2535.

2.      Wilson Zingg R, Kendall R. Obesity, Vascular Disease, and Lumbar Disk Degeneration: Associations of Comorbidities in Low Back Pain. PM R. 2016.

3.      Seyithanoglu H, Aydin T, Taspinar O, et al. Association between nutritional status and Modic classification in degenerative disc disease. J Phys Ther Sci. 2016;28(4):1250-1254.

# 22. MUSCLE PAIN

Myofascial pain is the most common form of musculoskeletal pain. Myofascial trigger points play an important role in the clinical manifestation of myofascial pain syndrome. Elucidating the role of central sensitization in the pathophysiology of trigger points is fundamental to developing optimal strategies in the management of myofascial pain syndrome.[1]

A myofascial pain syndrome is a soft tissue disorder of your muscles that can cause you not only to have pain for a long time, but it can also cause you to on occasion, have some disability. Your overall activities of daily living, including work, recreation and social interaction can be significantly affected.

Myofascial pain is pain related to muscle injury or overuse resulting in taut bands and palpable areas of pain that is referred to other muscular areas of your body. The pain can be dull, sharp or burning. You may suffer from sleep deprivation depression and anxiety like fibromyalgia. Your doctor may make a diagnosis of myofascial pain if you cry out or wince and withdraw away from light palpation on an area of your body

Muscle strains and ligament sprains can cause pain in your muscles and can contribute to the onset of a myofascial pain syndrome. The pain intensity of myofascial disorders can vary from painless decreases in range of motion about your arms, legs, neck, and lower back, which are common in older individuals, to pain that is agonizing and incapacitating.

Most myofascial pain can be relieved with an appropriate diagnosis and specific treatment. Pressing on the tender spots on your body can identify myofascial trigger points. When you tender area is pressed, you will have pain in other areas of your body that are away from the area being examined. Fibromyalgia pain does not cause referred pain when tender areas are palpated.

The pains in the other areas are referred pain patterns that demonstrate trigger points. Myofascial trigger points occur when there is trauma to your muscle or prolonged tension on your muscle from slouching over a desk or slouching over a worktable. This slouching results in disruption of your muscle cells.

When your muscle cell becomes disrupted, your cells release calcium. Calcium released inside of your muscle cell stimulates more contractions of your muscle. A prolonged contraction will exceed the available oxygen, glucose, and other nutrients that are needed for the energy to allow your muscle to continue to contract. With a sustained contraction, you run out of oxygen as well as other nutrients. This allows your muscle cell to build up a substance called lactic acid which stimulates muscle pain fibers.

Substances that cause your body to produce pain-causing substances are prostaglandins that sensitize pain fibers or substance P (a pain neuro-transmitter) that is involved in pin transmission. These pain transmitters then stimulate nerve endings around your muscle cells. These nerve endings go to other structures in your body. This is why you notice a referred pain pattern when you have a myofascial pain syndrome.

You will notice nodular, ropelike bands under your painful muscles when you have myofascial pain syndrome. The lack of oxygen in your muscle tissue will cause some of your muscle cells to die. This will cause scar tissue to form about your muscles. This scar tissue gives you the nodular feeling when you press over these painful areas.

Not all pain in your muscles is from myofascial pain. Sometimes ar-thritis can cause muscle pain surrounding your joints. Myopathy is a disease of muscles that can occur and cause you to have muscle pain. If you have a disc herniation, you can have referred pain to your muscles as well. Rocky Mountain Spotted-Fever or Lyme disease can also cause you to have muscle pain. A myofascial trigger point in your muscle needs to be distinguished from tender areas around your ligaments as well as around your bone.

The diagnosis of your myofascial pain syndrome is made by your health-care provider's history and physical examination and expertise. No laboratory tests are useful for the diagnosis of this syndrome. If you have the myofascial pain syndrome, you will complain of localized muscle pain and tenderness as well as the referred pain. If you have myofascial trigger points around your head and neck, you may com-plain of headaches as well as problems with your vision. Remember that you can have myofascial trigger points in one muscle or many muscles.

To make a diagnosis of myofascial trigger points, you must have painful areas in a muscle that is noted by your doctor on physical examina-tion. These painful areas must be nodular and must be reproducible.

Different amounts of pressure from your examining health-care pro-vider will give you referred pain. If you truly have myofascial pain your doctor will record whether you have a "jump sign" noted on physical exami-nation. This means that when your doctor applies pressure on your trigger point, you jump away from the pressure.

Your health-care provider will usually notice a twitch about the area that has pressure applied to it. At the time of your examination, your health care provided will notice that your pain diminishes with stretching or following injection of your muscle with a local anesthetic.

Your trigger points are classified as either active or latent. Active trigger points occur following acute muscle trauma. The latent trigger point on the other hand does not cause you to have pain at rest but can cause you to have restriction of movement about a certain part of your body. Latent trigger points are from a previous muscle injury. A latent trigger point can persist for years after recovery from an injury. Latent trigger points can predispose you to have pain with overuse of your previously injured muscle. Sometimes in cold weather, your muscle will contract and cause you to have pain.

Remember, only the active trigger points cause pain. The latent trigger points cause pain when they become active. Normal muscles do not have trigger points that can be felt or have areas that can cause you pain when touched. You should feel your normal muscles. Normal muscles do not have ropelike, nodular areas or tender areas to pressure and exhibit no observable twitch when your health-care provider palpates your muscle. Furthermore, you will not have referred pain with this applied pressure.

You can have different degrees of severity of myofascial pain. Some trigger points are much more sensitive than others. An extremely sensitive trigger point can cause you to have greater referred nerve pain than a less-severe or intense trigger point. Myofascial pain is usually not symmetrical on either side of your body. However, medical conditions that cause muscle pain such as fibromyalgia are symmetrical.

Trigger points are usually activated by overuse of muscles. You can stretch your muscle beyond its normal capability, which will cause your muscle to become injured. Bleeding can occur within your muscle following injury, which may cause scar formation in your muscle.

Active trigger points can develop in your muscles following excessive, repetitive, or sustained motions. For example, if you work in a warehouse and load heavy boxes all day over months, you can begin to develop active trigger points. Common areas of trigger point pain include your neck, arms, shoulders, face, back and legs.

Emotional stress can cause your muscles to stay in a contracted state. When your muscles are contracted for a length of time as previously stated, you lose oxygen and other nutrients to your muscle tissues. You must attempt to relax and do breathing exercises and range-of-motion exercises to decrease your pain. Heat and cold my help decrease your pain.

Myofascial pain can vary in pain severity from hour by hour or from day by day. If you do not exercise and do aerobic activity and are under a lot of stress, you have susceptibility to develop active trigger points.

Viral illnesses can cause muscle pain. If you have a virus, do not put cold packs on your muscles. A virus will activate chemicals in your body that activate pain signals. That is why you ache all over your body when you have the flu.

Myofascial pain may outlast any precipitating traumatic musculoskeletal event. The pain duration is of myofascial pain is longer in duration than the muscle strain duration. The duration depends on your overall muscular prior to an injury. If you are a professional football player for example, you can have a muscle strain and never develop trigger points. If you are not physically fit, a minor muscle strain can result in myfascial pain. A problem occurs when you are injured, your muscles have developed a way of trying to prevent further pain. In doing so, these other muscles will cause your injured muscle to be protected.

Eventually your active trigger points will become latent. If you rest your muscle and use a splint or an elastic bandage, your active trigger point may revert to become a latent trigger point. Occasionally you may do an activity that will activate your latent trigger point. This not unusual and you should expect this occurrence on occasion. Many of your muscles around your active trigger point can decrease their function, causing your muscles to become weak. If enough of your muscles lose a significant portion of their function, you can develop weakness of an entire extremity.

Myofascial pain is caused by pressure over your muscles. When you are lying in bed, you may have some pressure on your body in the area of the trigger points from your mattress. This pressure from your bed can cause you to have pain. On the other hand, be aware that sleep disturbances can cause your muscles to contract and become stiff and can worsen your myofascial pain syndrome.

There are no blood tests that will show abnormalities that can be attributed to a myofascial pain syndrome. X-rays, MRI images, and CAT scans have not demonstrated any changes that can be associated with myofascial trigger points either active or latent. There have been no reported electromyographic (EMG) changes when you have a myofascial pain syndrome.

The highest incidence of the onset of trigger points occurs between ages 31 and 50. When you are over 50, maximum activity could cause you to suffer from myofascial pain. As you continue to age and reduce your activity as a result of pain, your range of motion as a result of latent trigger points will become manifest. Many health-care providers are aware of myofascial trigger points.

Chiropractors treat myofascial trigger points, as do physical therapists. acupuncturists, anesthesiologists, dentists, pediatricians, rheumatologists, and specialists in physical medicine and rehabilitation all treat myofascial pain syndrome. The manner in which each of these health-care providers treats myofascial pain will vary from each of the health-care provider specialties.

If your pain is not relieved with conservative measures another method that can decrease your pain is a botulism toxin injection into your painful muscles. This drug is a gram-negative bacterium. In small doses it can relax or even paralyze small muscle fibers. The relief from the injection of the Botox can last up to three months. The problem with the Botox injection is that some individuals develop what appears to be fever and generalized joint pain associated with the bacteria that gets into their bloodstream. These side effects should however, subside over several days.

Given that no two people are alike, if you are taking any medications and begin to take nutritional supplements you should be aware that potential drug-nutrient interactions may occur and are encouraged to consult a health care professional before using any natural product. Combining certain prescription drugs and dietary supplements can lead to undesirable effects such as: diminished prescription drug effectiveness, reduced supplement effectiveness and impaired drug and/or supplement absorption.

Prevention of myofascial trigger points should be considered. This may be accomplished by doing stretching exercises both before and immediately after engaging in strenuous exercise. This concept may also be used if you are not physically fit and want to work in your garden for example. Do stretching exercises both before and after gardening. This may prevent the onset of myofascial pain.

Nutritional disorders have been reported to be important causal factors that can intensify or cause a painful response in individuals with chronic musculoskeletal pain. Patients with chronic myofascial pain showed lower intracellular stores of zinc and selenium and inadequate food intake of these nutrients.[2] Nutritional disorders have been reported to be important causal factors that can intensify or cause a painful response in individuals with chronic musculoskeletal pain.[3]

There also appears to be insufficient experimental data demonstrating ingestion of a protein supplement following a bout of exercise attenuates muscle soreness and/or lowers markers of muscle damage. However, beneficial effects such as reduced muscle soreness and markers of muscle damage become more evident when supplemental protein is consumed after daily training sessions.[4]

Reference

1.      Srbely JZ, Dickey JP, Bent LR, Lee D, Lowerison M. Capsaicin-induced central sensitization evokes segmental increases in trigger point sensitivity in humans. J Pain. 2010;11(7):636-643.

2.      Hutchins MO, Feine JS. Neuromuscular dysfunction: the role of nutrition. Compend Contin Educ Dent. 1985;6(1):38-39, 42-35.

3.      Barros-Neto JA, Souza-Machado A, Kraychete DC, et al. Selenium and Zinc Status in Chronic Myofascial Pain: Serum and Erythrocyte Concentrations and Food Intake. PLoS One. 2016;11(10):e0164302.

4.      Pasiakos SM, Lieberman HR, McLellan TM. Effects of protein supplements on muscle damage, soreness and recovery of muscle function and physical performance: a systematic review. Sports Med. 2014;44(5):655-670.

Fibromyalgia is a chronic pain syndrome that affects muscles, tendons, and fascia (a tissue area over your muscle) throughout your body. This disease is also referred to as fibromyositis. It affects about 5 percent of the population, 90 percent of which are women of childbearing age. You and your physician must function together as a team to properly treat this entity. Fibromyalgia causes you to have muscle pain through-out your body, and is associated with joint stiffness and fatigue.

You also may experience sleep disturbances and depression if you have fibromyalgia. It can cause many places on your body to become extremely tender. You are only diagnosed with fibromyalgia after other pain-causing conditions have been eliminated as the reason for your pain. Fibromyalgia is a condition that can be painful, but it is benign and will rarely cause you to be totally disabled. Only you can let it become disabling.

The diagnosis of fibromyalgia includes a history of aches, pains, stiffness in 11 or more tender areas above and below your navel and to the right and left of your navel (figure 1). You may have a history of irritable bowel syndrome and depression as well. You may be de-pressed and suffer from sleep deprivation in addition to muscle pain. In 2010, the American College of Rheumatology published a new set of preliminary guidelines. These guidelines include a widespread pain index that assesses the number of painful body regions, and a scale that assesses the severity of symptoms such as fatigue, sleep problems, comprehension problems, and others in the body.

By using one or both of these sets of guidelines, along with tests to rule out other possible conditions, it is possible for your doctor to make a fibromyalgia diagnosis.

The following diagram shows common body sites where you might experience tender areas associated with fibromyalgia. You muscle will not feel contracted but will feel soft and tender to light touch. Tender areas can also occur in your arms and legs. You should note from the diagram that these tender points occur above and below your navel and occur in a plane to the right and left of your navel.

If you are like other patients with fibromyalgia, the muscle pain that you experience is probably more common in your neck and lower back. However, it can affect any muscle throughout your body. Your pain can range from sharp or cramping to a burning sensation. Your pain may be worse in one specific area, even though the pain can be felt all over your body. You also will notice that fibromyalgia pain affects tender areas on your body that are symmetrical, or located in the same places on the opposite side of your body.

Tenderness and swelling of your hands or feet are also common. Other common areas where you may notice tenderness include the areas under the base of your skull; above the shoulder blade, elbows, the buttocks (gluteal muscle); the front of the neck midway from the chin to the collar bone; the chest; the sides of the body over the hip regions; and the inner aspects of the knees.

It is more common for women to have fibromyalgia than men. Because of this, researchers are trying to find gender-specific causes of fibromyalgia. In general the amount of pain that women can withstand is lower than the amount of pain that men can withstand. Fibromyalgia is seen mostly in women between 20 and 50 years of age. However, it can affect children and elderly people as well.

Fibromyalgia may develop after an injury, a motor vehicle accident, infection (viral or bacterial), or after an onset of rheumatoid arthritis. Stressful situations, cold weather and over exertion can worsen your fibromyalgia. As a fibromyalgia sufferer, you may not be getting enough deep sleep. Even in normal people, not getting enough sleep can produce symptoms of fibromyalgia. It is not currently known if a lack of deep sleep is a cause of fibromyalgia. Some doctors think the loss of deep sleep can hasten the onset of fibromyalgia.

Serotonin and norepinepherine are two chemicals in your central nervous system (brain and spinal cord) that decrease pain signals that travel to your brain. Not having enough serotonin in your brain and spinal cord can cause you lose sleep, which can cause symptoms of depression as well as fibromyalgia like pain. Fibromyalgia also affects your levels of norepinepherine, which is another chemical in your central nervous that also modulates the number of pain signals that go to your brain. Another chemical in your body that causes pain is substance P.

Substance P is found in all of the neurons of your central nervous system as well as nerves that go to your muscles and joints. When your muscle tissues have been injured, substance P is released. This event can trigger burning pain sensations throughout your body. High substance P levels have been noted in the spinal fluid of patients with fibromyalgia. Endorphins, substances produced by your body and deposited in the spinal cord to decrease pain transmission to your brain, are known to slow down the pain-causing effects of substance P. The low levels of endorphins in your brain and spinal cord when you have fibromyalgia may be another cause of pain associated with this condition.

It is well known that vigorous exercise can produce endorphins that are then released in your body. Along with decreasing the pain signals that are sent to your brain, endorphins can affect your mood. It is thought that a lower than normal blood level of endorphins may be another cause of fibromyalgia. People with and without fibromyalgia who do physical exercise have noted a decrease in their pain following aerobic exercise. Normal people usually have an increase in endorphins in their bloodstream following exercise. However, you may show no increase in endorphin levels after you exercise.

There is increased evidence that fibromyalgia can be genetically inherited. You may even know of a relative who has symptoms similar to yours. The exact gene that causes fibromyalgia has not been isolated, but several genes have been proposed as a possible explanation for the genetic inheritance of fibromyalgia and they are being studied. Research into the causes of fibromyalgia must continue.

It is a good idea for you to keep a daily diary of your activities and pain levels. When you visit your doctor, be sure to take your diary with you so your doctor can see your daily activities such as exercise, sleep, and eating habits. Also be sure to write down any medications you have taken and what their effects were. This will help your doctor determine what areas you need help in the most, and can help the doctor prescribe an effective treatment to relieve your pain symptoms. Let your pain-management doctor know if your primary care doctor diagnosed any new disorder or prescribed any new drug since your last visit with your pain doctor.

It is important that you do exercise or some type of low-impact aerobic activity. Aerobic exercise is extremely helpful in decreasing your pain and improving your sleep pattern. Swimming and water aerobics are excellent ways for you to accomplish this goal. They are some of the best exercise activities for patients with fibromyalgia. These types of nonimpact activities will help strengthen and condition your muscles, unlike high-impact exercise that can actually do more damage to your muscles. A study published in 1996 said that following physical exercise, almost 50 percent of people had a significant decrease in their signs and symptoms of fibromyalgia. Exercise will improve your muscle range of motion.

Most doctors agree that medications, injections, and therapy alone will not be able to eliminate your pain, but rather it will help you to manage your pain and cope with it better. Taking steroids to treat your fibromyalgia will not improve your symptoms of pain. People with other muscle or bone conditions such as rheumatoid arthritis do respond well to steroids. However, nonsteroidal anti-inflammatory medications such as ibuprofen may relieve or at least decrease your muscle pain.

The primary goal in treating your fibromyalgia is to attempt to break the pain cycle. One way of accomplishing this goal is to correct any disturbance in your sleep pattern. Amitriptyline (Elavil) can be an important drug in restoring your sleep. Numerous studies have shown that getting enough sleep can significantly reduce your pain.

If you are allergic to amitriptyline, cyclobenzaprine (Flexeril) can be substituted. In some people, nonsteroidal anti-inflammatory medications such as ibuprofen can be successfully used. Amantadine hydrochloride (Symmetrel) also may be used. This medication is an antiviral as well as an anti-Parkinson medication. Serotonin reuptake inhibitors (Paxil) may also have a positive effect on reducing your pain. There are new two drugs approved by the FDA for the treatment of fibromyalgia; Lyrica (an anticonvulsant) and Cymbalta (an antidepressant). Savella or Celexa may also be helpful.

Nerve stimulation is another method of relieving pain that you may find helpful. A TENS unit (Transcutaneous Electrical Nerve Stimulator) is useful in managing fibromyalgia pain in many patients. This small battery-powered instrument has two to four patches that are placed over your painful muscle areas. Electrical impulses will stimulate the nerves around your areas of pain. This stimulation will cause the production of the pain-relieving chemical enkephalin into your spinal cord. Enkephalin will diminish the intensity of your pain signals that ultimately reach your brain.

Another useful device that is gaining in popularity is a muscle stimula-tor. This device has six to eight patches that are placed over your painful muscle areas. The muscle stimulator machine will stimulate and work your muscles until they are fatigued and weakened. It is possible for your muscles that have been weakened by the fibromyalgia to be strengthened this way.

Be aware of the "leaking gut" theory as a cause of fibromyalgia. If large proteins leak into your gastrointestinal circulation, your immune system may become overactive. You can then experience an antibody response that causes you to have generalized body pain. Some individuals that have fibromyalgia from this cause can be treated successfully with a gluten free diet, colostrums supplements or hyperimmune eggs.

A psychologist can help you deal with the suffering aspect of your pain. Your psychologist also may want to teach you biofeedback. This is a good way for you to learn relaxing techniques that can significantly reduce your pain. Your psychologist may want you to listen to a CD or cassette tapes at home. Aromatherapy also could be effective for helping you manage your pain. This method is more effective in women because their scent perception is better than a man's. You may also find that hypnosis can decrease your pain intensity as well. You may want to try self-hypnosis as another modality for the management of your chronic pain.

Insomina is common in fibromyalgia. Chronic insomnia alone impacts 10% to 15% of adults. Epidemiologic data indicate that pain, fatigue, and mood disturbance are common correlates of persistent insomnia. Your physician must try to correct your insomnia. A good night's rest increases norepinerpherine and serotonin in your central nervous system. These are two biochemicals that can decrease your pain.

Given that no two people are alike, if you are taking any medications and begin to take nutritional supplements you should be aware that potential drug-nutrient interactions may occur and are encouraged to consult a health care professional before using any natural product. Combining certain prescription drugs and dietary supplements can lead to undesirable effects such as: diminished prescription drug effectiveness, reduced supplement effectiveness and impaired drug and/or supplement absorption.

Coenzyme Q10 (CoQ10) deficiency has been implicated in the pathophysiology of fibromyalgia. All patients in one study with fibromyalgia showed CoQ10 deficiency.[1] After treatment, all patients showed an important improvement in clinical symptoms in all evaluation methods. According to these results, and evaluated by three methods, patients with FM are candidates for treatment with CoQ10.

Many people suffer from fibromyalgia (FM) without an effective treatment. They do not have a good quality of life and cannot maintain normal daily activity. Vegetarian diets could have some beneficial effects probably due to the increase in antioxidant intake.[2]

The results of a pilot study suggest that dietary Chlorella supplementation may help relieve the symptoms of fibromyalgia in some patients.[3] Moreover, it seems reasonable to eliminate some foods from the diet of FM patients, for example excitotoxins. Non-celiac gluten sensitivity is increasingly recognized as a frequent condition with similar manifestations which overlap with those of FM.[4] The elimination of gluten from the diet of FM patients is recently becoming a potential dietary intervention for clinical improvement.

References

1.     Alcocer-Gomez E, Cano-Garcia FJ, Cordero MD. Effect of coenzyme Q10 evaluated by 1990 and 2010 ACR Diagnostic Criteria for

Fibromyalgia and SCL-90-R: four case reports and literature review. Nutrition. 2013;29(11-12):1422-1425.

2.        Arranz LI, Canela MA, Rafecas M. Fibromyalgia and nutrition, what do we know? Rheumatol Int. 2010;30(11):1417-1427.

3.        Merchant RE, Carmack CA, Wise CM. Nutritional supplementation with Chlorella pyrenoidosa for patients with fibromyalgia syndrome: a pilot study. Phytother Res. 2000;14(3):167-173.

4.        Rossi A, Di Lollo AC, Guzzo MP, et al. Fibromyalgia and nutrition: what news? Clin Exp Rheumatol. 2015;33(1 Suppl 88):S117-125.

# 24. HEADACHES

Headaches can have many causes. Most headaches are caused by emotional stress or fatigue, but some headaches are a symptom of a disease within the brain. Of the many pains that you can feel through-out your body, pain in the head region is usually the most distressing. Pain in your head can arise in your head itself or can be referred from your neck as well.

There are two general classes of headaches, primary and secondary. Primary headaches are those that occur from structures within your brain while secondary headaches can be caused by tumors, infections, etc. Primary headaches have no structural, infectious or other abnormality that could cause your headache. Examples of primary head-aches are migraine head-aches and tension-type headaches. Secondary headaches have underlying abnormalities like a tumor, hemorrhage, blood clot, etc.

Some pain receptors exist outside your skull, and other pain receptors exist within your skull. Structures outside of your skull that can cause pain in your head include the skin and scalp over your head, muscles about your head and neck, and the outer wrapper of the bone of your skull called the periosteum.

Your sinuses can also cause you to have head pain immediately above your eyes. Within your skull, you have a lining that can become inflamed and irritated and cause pain called the meninges. Your veins can cause pain as well if they become engorged. You must tell your doctor where the location of your pain is. This will help your doctor determine the source of your headache.

Your doctor will complete a detailed history and neurological examination and may order a MRI or CAT scan to determine what type of headache that you have. The purpose of a neurological examination is to exclude any disease or tumor outside of your brain that could be causing your headache. If you have a history of rheumatoid arthritis, make sure that your doctor knows that you have this disorder. Headaches can arise from instability of the first two bones in your neck.

Because tight muscles can also cause headaches, your doctor will check the muscles in your neck. Your doctor will then press on the arteries in your temples. If you have tenderness around the arteries in your temples, you may have an inflammation of your temporal arteries. This disease is called temporal arteritis. Your doctor will have you lie flat on the examining table. Your doctor will ask whether you have a change in your headache after your head is lifted. If your headache is originating from your neck, there may be some relief by lifting your head relative to your neck.

Skull X-rays can prove useful for the diagnosis of a skull fracture, cancers, bone destruction, or some shift of the structures of the brain. If you have pain in your neck, your doctor may order x-rays of your neck, with your neck bent forward and then bent backward.

This is called a flexion-extension X ray. This test can determine whether you have any instability of the bones in your neck. Blood flow studies may be done to determine whether you have any compromise in the blood flow going to your brain. A decrease in blood flow can cause significant headaches.

Sometimes a CT scan is necessary to determine whether you have swelling in your brain or a brain abscess. An electroencephalogram (EEG) study is sometimes ordered to determine whether you have a seizure disorder or a sleep problem. If you have had trauma to your head, your doctor may want a CAT scan, which will show whether you have bleeding within your head.

An MRI scan of your brain can be done to see whether you have loss of myelin, which is a substance in your brain. With loss of myelin, you may develop neurological symptoms that include memory loss and difficulty concentrating and have pain in your legs. This disease is called Multiple Sclerosis.

Occasionally a spinal tap is done to help make a diagnosis of what may be causing your headache. This procedure can investigate whether you have an infection such as meningitis. This procedure consists of placing a needle into your spinal fluid. At the time that the spinal tap is done, a pressure monitor can be used to see whether you have increased pressure in your central nervous system.

Be aware, that the medical history that you give to your doctor is important. Do not leave out any information. Information that is not important to you may be very important to your physician. Your doctor needs to know if you have had a headache with loss of consciousness. Loss of consciousness could indicate seizures or a hemorrhage into your brain.

If you have had no previous history of a severe headache, your doctor may need to order tests to see whether or not you have a bleed in your brain from a weakness in one of the arteries (aneurysm) in your brain. A weakness in the blood vessel is called an aneurysm. If you have headaches accompanied by neurological abnormalities during and after your headache, your doctor will want to make sure that you do not have a clot within your brain or a brain tumor.

Tumors can cause headaches with neurological abnormalities such as forgetfulness and dizziness. If you have a headache that first begins after age 50, your pain may be coming from degeneration of the discs in your neck. Hormonal changes that can occur with decreased function of your thyroid gland can cause headaches as well.

Depression also can also cause headaches. If someone has told you that your personality changes when you have a headache, your doctor will want to determine whether you have a tumor or even an infection of your brain.

A headache that occurs when you have an increase in your blood pressure can indicate various medical diseases that may be causing a headache. Be aware that headaches can come from the soft tissues in your neck. An x-ray of your neck will not reveal soft tissue problems. An MRI can usually reveal problems in structures that could cause you to have a headache.

A common type of headache is the classic migraine headache. By definition a migraine headache is a headache that returns and varies widely in its intensity and frequency of the attacks and the duration. Usually the headaches occur on one side and are associated with nausea, vomiting, and a loss of appetite. Sometimes you may have visual problems associated with this headache. You can have a head-ache with sensations that forewarn you of an attack of an impending headache.

You may have a sensation of flickering lights or blurred vision or weakness in your arms or legs. These sensations are called an aura. Some migraines occur without an aura. If you have migraines with an aura, usually you have visual disturbances. This type of visual disturb-ance is seen in 90 percent of patients who have migraine headaches with an aura. Migraine headaches can be triggered if you have abnormal response to stress. No one knows what exactly causes migraine headaches. When you have one of these headaches, you may experience mood disturbances as well as pain. You may have nausea and vomiting as well.

Migraine headaches usually begin when you are a teenager. However, some migraine headaches can begin at age 40. Before you suffer a migraine headache, you may have changes in your vision or speech and balance. You may notice zigzag lines in front of your eyes or small specks in one eye.

You may notice different lines that come and go in front of your eyes. You may have numbness in your hands. When the headache occurs following these visual disturbances, your headache is usually on one side of your head.

If you are seeing lines only in front of your left eye, usually your headache will be on the right side of your brain. Sometimes you can have migraine headaches that occur several times a week followed by a long period of having no headaches. Sometimes your migraine headaches can be incapacitating. Movements such as bending over, coughing or sneezing can worsen your headache. You will want to lie down. Following your headache, it can take approximately 24 hours for you to feel normal again.

If you have a history of migraine headaches, be aware that some stressful situations such as weddings, funerals, or speaking in front of people can trigger a migraine headache. Be aware that there can be a family history of migraine headaches. Seventy percent of people inherit the tendency to have migraine headaches. If you have migraine headaches, you usually have less than two attacks per month. However, 10 percent of patients have attacks every week.

Some migraine headaches begin with a visual aura of zigzag lines or a blotting out of your vision or both. Furthermore, numbness of one side of your face and hand, weakness, unsteadiness, or altered conscious-ness may precede your headache. Most however, are not associated with an aura. The aura can forewarn you of an impending headache. This type of headache is called a migraine headache without an aura. Sometimes these headaches occur on both sides of your head but most occur on just one side of your head.

Before your doctor prescribes medicines for your headache, your doctor must tailor your medications to your type of headache and take into account your disability, your medical history, and your psychological profile. Treatment of your migraines can be divided into acute treatment of the attack as well as treatment to prevent the onset of headaches. Whenever possible, the factors that cause your headaches should be avoided. Stay away from foods that could trigger your migraine head-ache. Cheese, chocolate, red wine, and some Chinese foods that contain the additive MSG are commonly considered migraine headache triggers.

If you have an onset of a headache, a mild attack can be treated with aspirin. Nonsteroidal anti-inflammatory drugs can also be used to treat your headache. Ibuprofen is commonly used to treat headaches and can be purchased without a prescription. The nonsteroidal anti-inflammatory drugs called COX-2 inhibitors (Celebrex) can also be effective for the treatment of headaches. If you have nausea and vomiting associated with your migraine headache, you may need to take a nonsteroidal anti-inflammatory drug by the rectal route.

Newer drugs called triptans have been developed and can decrease your headache within a significant time after its onset. Sumatriptan was the first triptan drug to be used for the treatment of migraine headaches. Triptans are much better tolerated than the older caffeine-ergotamine medications. Be aware that the triptans are expensive. When you first suspect that you are having a migraine, take your triptan immediately.

Sometimes stronger drugs are needed for the treatment of migraine headache symptoms. Codeine is sometimes needed. Stronger drugs such as Percocet have been prescribed for the treatment of migraine headaches. If you have frequent migraine attacks and if these attacks are disabling, your physician may consider prophylactic treatment. Because migraine headaches can be activated by stress, it is important that you tell your doctor what situations trigger your head-aches.

You may have to make life adjustments to control your headaches. If you are having too much stress at work, you may need to consider changing your job. If you have significant psychological problems, consider a consultation with a psychologist. Antihypertensive medications such as Nadolol and Verapamil have been used to prevent the onset of migraine headaches. Amitriptyline, an antidepressant, also has been demonstrated to prevent the onset of migraine headache.

Migraine headaches can be hormonally related in females. They are more common in women until age 60 when the incidence is about equal with men. Migraine headaches commonly occur with the onset of menses in women. These headaches may also occur in the first trimester of pregnancy. The headaches can disappear following a complete hysterectomy.

After the onset of menopause, your migraine headaches may disappear or at least decrease in intensity and frequency. However, if you receive hormone therapy at the time of menopause, this can prolong your headache symptoms.

Sometimes your migraine headaches can worsen when you begin using oral contraceptives. Concern exists about the use of oral contraceptives by those who suffer migraine headaches, because they run a higher risk of stroke.

Another type of headache that you could experience is called a tension-type headache. This also is called a muscle contraction headache even though muscle tightness is not a common cause of this type of headache. If you have chronic tension-type headaches, you may have headaches 15 days a month. For your doctor to make a diagnosis of your tension-type headache, you should have at least 10 previous headache episodes.

The headaches could last from 30 minutes to 7 days. You will usually have a headache on both sides of your head. Your headaches should not be aggravated by walking or routine physical activity. If you have a tension-type headache, you should not experience nausea or vomiting. You should not have visual disturbances that are associated with migraine headaches.

Migraine headaches and tension-type headaches are experienced more in women than men. Muscle tension-type headaches can start at any age. Tension-type headaches can begin in childhood if a child is physically and emotionally abused. When you have a tension-type headache, you will feel a tight band and pressure around your head in the form of a tight cap. Your neck muscles will feel as if they are in a knot. The location of your pain is usually all around your head on both sides. Usually a tension-type headache is seen in tense or anxious people.

If depression perpetuates your headaches, you can take antidepressants at bedtime to enhance your sleep or take an antidepressant like Cymbalta during the day. Sometimes muscle relaxants can be used to decrease your pain. Antianxiety drugs such as Valium have sometimes been used preventatively to decrease the chance of one of these headaches developing. When your headache occurs, one of the nonsteroidal anti-inflammatory drugs may be helpful in decreasing your headache.

Another type of headache that you should be aware of is called a cluster headache. This severely painful headache is not common and occurs mostly in men. Usually the headache is on one side of your head and can be above your eye or in your temple. Usually the headache lasts 15 minutes to 3 hours if untreated.

Usually you will have tearing of your eye as well as nasal congestion on the side of your cluster headache. You may have forehead sweating. Your pupil may be extremely small and your upper eyelid may droop. These headaches can be extremely painful. The exact cause of cluster headaches is unknown.

A cluster headache occurs more frequently in men than in women. They also occur more frequently in the spring and fall and occur at the same time of the day. There is a 5:1 man-to-woman ratio of cluster headaches. To treat a cluster headache attack, some doctors suggest inhalation of 100 percent oxygen using a face mask.

Usually your headache will settle in 15 minutes. If this does not work, an injection of sumatriptan (Imitrex) may decrease your pain. Some studies have even recommended the use of local anesthetics on a cotton swab placed in your nose.

Steroids in high doses can be used to treat cluster headaches. Medrol (a steroid) can be given in various doses and schedules as directed by your treating physician. This drug must be discontinued slowly after treatment for five to seven days. It may take up to three weeks to taper the drug. Non-steroidal anti-inflammatory drugs may be effective in the treatment of these headaches as well. Sometimes sufferers need to see a neurosurgeon in consultation to see whether there is a surgical procedure that can be done to decrease the frequency of these headaches.

A headache following trauma can be made worse with physical exercise. A post-traumatic headache differs from migraine symptoms in that a chronic post-traumatic headache is usually generalized and permanent. However, it can be made worse by physical or mental strain. Usually this type of headache subsides in 8 to 10 weeks.

You can develop a post-traumatic headache with only a minor injury to your head. In fact, the more severe the injury, the less chance you have of developing one of these headaches. Post-traumatic headache is reported more often in women than men. The incidence of a post-traumatic headache can be forty percent following a head injury.

If you are over 60 years of age, you could develop a headache related to temporal arteritis. This usually occurs after you have had a fever. You have a burning pain caused by inflammation of your temporal artery on the side of your head. It is usually accompanied by a throbbing headache about your temple.

With temporal arteritis you may have a burning pain about your scalp. Jaw movement such as chewing worsens temporal arteritis headaches. This type of headache can be accompanied by loss of vision, which is a medical emergency. The diagnosis sometimes has to be made with a biopsy of the arterial tissue. Steroids are usually the treatment of choice for this pain.

Pain in your head can come from direct pressure on structures such as nerves, muscles or blood vessels. Traction on your nerves can cause your pain. If your blood vessels become engorged and if the diameters of your vessels become enlarged, the enlarged vessel can compress your nerves in your brain and cause you to have a headache. A prolonged muscle contraction in your neck can cause pain as well.

Psychological distress can trigger your headaches. Sometimes major social trauma or anxiety triggers headaches. Physical trauma can also be a cause of chronic headaches. If you are a woman, your doctor will want to know the effects of your menstrual periods and pregnancy on your headaches.

enstrual periods and pregnancies change hormones in the bloodstream, and this change can trigger headaches. Hormone changes in both men and women can increase you incidence of headaches.

A headache that begins at the base of your skull is called occipital neuralgia. The pain from occipital neuralgia shoots up to the top of your head. Local pressure on the back of your head will reproduce your pain. Trauma to the back of your head or an infection can cause pain. Degeneration disc disease may also cause occipital neuralgia. Your do
           ctor may order a CAT scan to try and determine what is causing your pain. Treatment may consist of muscle relaxants, non-steroidal anti-inflammatory drugs, and antidepressant drugs, injections with steroids, botulism toxin or local anesthetics. On occasion, freezing the Greater Occipital nerve may relieve your pain. Currently treatment with a peripheral electrical stimulating wire is gaining popularity.

It appears that there is gender specificity with respect to headaches. In men, when their testosterone increases, cluster headaches become frequent. Cluster headaches are can occur at the onset of puberty. In males and females with an increase in progesterone, estrogen, and testosterone, there is an increase in migraine as well as tension headaches.

Be aware that women produce testosterone as well as men. When progesterone, estrogen, and testosterone blood levels increase in your body, pain in general increases in both men and women.

In many instances physicians are under the misconception that a detailed biochemical understanding of each individual disease is required before nutritional interventions can be used. Natural remedy is cheap, easily available, nontoxic, and easy to prepare and provides good mental health as compared to other remedies.

A moderate dose of caffeine can also help relieve a headache (especially the type that cause throbbing or pounding) by constricting the blood vessels that go to the head.

Given that no two people are alike, if you are taking any medications and begin to take nutritional supplements you should be aware that potential drug-nutrient interactions may occur and are encouraged to consult a health care professional before using any natural product.

Combining certain prescription drugs and dietary supplements can lead to undesirable effects such as: diminished prescription drug effectiveness, reduced supplement effectiveness and impaired drug and/or supplement absorption.

Omega-3 and omega-6 fatty acids are precursors of bioactive lipid mediators posited to modulate both physical pain and psychological distress.

In a randomized trial of 67 subjects with severe headaches, it was demonstrated that targeted dietary manipulation-increasing omega-3 fatty acids with concurrent reduction in omega-6 linoleic acid produced major reductions in headaches compared with an omega-6 lowering intervention alone.[1]

Riboflavin is a safe and well-tolerated option for preventing migraine symptoms in adults.2 Dietary sodium may affect brain extracellular fluid sodium concentrations and neuronal excitability.[3]

Another study demonstrated a harmful association between excess dietary salt and all-cause mortality, noncardiovascular and cardiovascular disease mortality, and headache.[4]

It has also been shown that Vitamin D supplementation may be useful in decreasing frequency of headache attacks.[5] The ability of CoQ(10) to mitigate headache symptoms in adults has also verified in pediatric and adolescent populations.[6]

Based on a nationally representative sample, it was found that cigarette smoking was associated with headache in an exposure-response manner. Mentholated cigarette smokers were not more likely to have headache compared to non-mentholated cigarette smokers.[7]

References

1.      Ramsden CE, Faurot KR, Zamora D, et al. Targeted alterations in dietary n-3 and n-6 fatty acids improve life functioning and reduce psychological distress among patients with chronic headache: a secondary analysis of a randomized trial. Pain. 2015;156(4):587-596.

2.      Namazi N, Heshmati J, Tarighat-Esfanjani A. Supplementation with Riboflavin (Vitamin B2) for Migraine Prophylaxis in Adults and Children: A Review. Int J Vitam Nutr Res. 2015;85(1-2):79-87.

3.      Pogoda JM, Gross NB, Arakaki X, Fonteh AN, Cowan RP, Harrington MG. Severe Headache or Migraine History is Inversely Correlated With Dietary Sodium Intake: NHANES 1999-2004. Headache. 2016;56(4):688-698.

4.      Johnson C, Raj TS, Trieu K, et al. The Science of Salt: A Systematic Review of Quality Clinical Salt Outcome Studies June 2014 to May 2015. J Clin Hypertens (Greenwich). 2016;18(9):832-839.

5.      Mottaghi T, Askari G, Khorvash F, Maracy MR. Effect of Vitamin D supplementation on symptoms and C-reactive protein in migraine patients. J Res Med Sci. 2015;20(5):477-482.

6.      Littarru GP, Tiano L. Clinical aspects of coenzyme Q10: an update. Nutrition. 2010;26(3):250-254.

7.       Gan WQ, Estus S, Smith JH. Association Between Overall and Mentholated Cigarette Smoking With Headache in a Nationally Representative Sample. Headache. 2016;56(3):511-518.

A neuropathy is by definition, pathology (disease or injury) of a nerve or nerves that exist outside of your brain and spinal cord. These nerves are called peripheral nerves. A disease of any of these nerves can cause a weakness in the muscle that it goes to and may possibly cause numbness and pain in the areas to where the nerve travels. If only one nerve is affected it is called a mononeuropathy. A polyneuropathy involves more than one nerve. A momoneuropathy is usually related to a nerve compression while a polyneuropathy is usually caused by a disease like diabetes.

With the onset of a neuropathy you will feel a burning or stinging pain in the area of the affected nerve. Sometimes a slight touch of the skin over your diseased nerve can cause incapacitating pain. Your symptoms are usually individualized, which means that your symptoms may differ from other patient's symptoms with the same nerve pathology. For example, if the nerve in your wrist, the median nerve, is com-pressed by tissue, you can develop a carpal tunnel syndrome.

You may have numbness in the area of your wrist, whereas another person may complain of pain or numbness that radiates into his or her finger tips. As a result, the treatment that works best for you may not work for other people with the same type of neuropathy.

Any neuropathy may cause a burning, gnawing pain. You can have some decreased sensation about the painful nerve. Extreme pain from just light touch can occur in tissues over the nerve. You can have increased sweating, cold sensations, or skin discoloration in the extremity associated with a neuropathy.

The onset of your pain following an injury to your nerve can either be of an immediate onset or a delayed gradual onset over weeks to months. Not all neuropathies cause pain. Some neuropathies cause only numbness. Neuropathies are diagnosed by electromyography and nerve conduction tests.

Entrapment neuropathies such as the carpal tunnel syndrome are characterized by abnormal sensations in the area of the nerve as well as pain. For example, a band of tissue at your wrist can compress a nerve going to your hand and fingers that can result in weakness and pain in your hand.

You can have a neuropathy that is not painful but it can cause you to have abnormal feelings in the tissue around your injured nerve. This abnormality is called a paresthesia. You have probably heard of a Morton's neuralgia. This can cause a severe entrapment of the small nerves that are around the bones that make up the foot. You may have significant burning pain with this neuropathy.

Some drugs can cause neuropathies. For example, the drug Isonizid used for the treatment of tuberculosis can cause a neuropathy. Arsenic can also cause a neuropathy. Diseases can also cause neuropathies as well. You may develop a painful neuropathy related to chronic renal failure (kidney failure). In addition, people who suffer with the HIV or AIDS can have extremely debilitating neuropathies associated with their disease.

Cancers may also cause a neuropathy. Your malignancy can cause you to have a progressive sensory neuropathy that usually is not painful. You may develop weakness or numbness in one or several of your nerves.

Carpal tunnel syndrome starts gradually with aching in your wrist that can extend to your forearm. You will develop pins and needles in your hand and fingers. This sensation can occur while you are driving, holding a phone, or reading this book.

You may develop weakness in your hands and drop objects. The diagnosis of a carpal tunnel syndrome can be done by arthroscopy, which consists of putting a scope into your carpal tunnel or by a nerve conduction test. An MRI of your wrist and hand can be done as well. There are no blood tests that can detect a carpal tunnel syndrome.

The carpal tunnel is a narrow passage at your wrist about the diameter of your thumb. The purpose of this tunnel is to protect your median nerve as well as the tendons that go to your fingers. The problem is that excessive pressure on this nerve will cause you to have numbness and pain and can lead to hand weakness. Compression of the median nerve in the carpal tunnel is a common compression neuropathy.

A carpal tunnel syndrome affects women more than men. The average age of the onset of this ailment is between 40 and 60 years of age. This condition can be caused by any continuous repetitive movement of your hand, such as typing or working with a computer.

If you are obese, pregnant, have a decrease in your thyroid function, or have Raynaud's disease or diabetes or renal failure, you are at a higher risk of developing a carpal tunnel syndrome than the population in general.

When your health-care provider initially sees you, you will be treated with immobilization of your wrist with a splint. This will prevent pressure on your nerve. If this method fails, you will be given an anti-inflammatory drug or an injection of Cortisone into your carpal tunnel to decrease the swelling in your tendons and ligaments within the tunnel. If this method fails, you will be a candidate for surgery. Surgery to release the tissue that is compressing your median nerve has been shown to be effective for the treatment of carpal tunnel syndrome.

Another common condition that can cause a neuropathy is diabetes. Diabetes can be associated with a polyneuropathy, which means that many nerves are involved in the disease process. A low thyroid level can also be a cause of a neuropathy. If you develop polyneuropathy, it occurs usually on both sides of your body and usually in both lower extremities from the knees down to your feet. Numbness and abnormal sensations are the most frequent complaints associated with this neuropathy.

You can have complaints of burning pain ranging from mild to severe in both legs. On occasion you may have symptoms of pains that are described as sharp, bolting, shock-like pain. Because diabetes can cause you to have a decrease in blood flow to your feet, make sure that you wear proper fitting shoes. Poor fitting shoes can cause ulcers on the bottom of your feet.

Diabetes can cause multiple nerve disorders in your peripheral nerves.. However, some of the nerves coming off of your brain can transmit pain signals to your face and your diabetes can also adversely affect these nerves. This may cause you to have facial pain.

Not only can you develop pain in your legs, you can also develop weakness in your legs as a result of your diabetic neuropathy. Some individuals with a diabetic neuropathy can have constant pain. The type of diabetic neuropathy is called diabetic amyotrophy. This entity occurs on one side of your body. It occurs most often in the nerves that go to your muscles.

The nerves that go to your muscles are called motor nerves. The diabetic amyotrophy is a motor neuropathy. The diabetic amyotrophy neuropathy, as well as other diabetic neuropathies, can be seen if you have poor control over your diabetes. Diabetic neuropathies are found in middle-aged as well as elderly patients who suffer with diabetes.

Careful attention to control over blood sugar in the long term is the best way to prevent diabetic neuropathy. The treatment of painful diabetic neuropathy has included anticonvulsive medications such as Tegretol.

Neurontin has become more popular over the past several years. Lyrica is a newer drug that is approved for the treatment of a diabetic neuropathy. Tricyclic antidepressant drugs such as Elavil can help to relieve your pain.

An antidepressant drug called Cymbalta is approved for the treatment of diabetic neuropathy. A drug that has been used successfully for the treatment of a painful diabetic neuropathy is mexiletine. This drug is essentially a medication that is used if you have abnormal heartbeats. This drug has been shown to be effective for the treatment of your diabetic neuropathy as well.

You can anticipate a positive reaction to oral mexiletine if you are given intravenous Lidocaine and have pain relief with this drug. Lidocaine is not only a numbing medicine but it is also a drug used for irregular rhythms of your heart. If you have significant pain relief with the administration of mexiletine administered intravenously the chances are that you will have excellent relief with the oral mexiletine.

Excessive alcohol consumption can cause neuropathies. Approximately 20 percent of chronic alcoholics develop peripheral neuropathy related to their alcohol consumption. The neuropathy affects not only sensation but can affect muscle strength in your legs.

When alcohol con-sumption is discontinued the neuropathy can recover, but the recovery is slow. The alcoholic neuropathy is believed to be due to a deficiency of thiamine as well as other B vitamins. Tegretol or Neurontin or a tricyclic antidepressant such as Elavil can also be used for the treatment of this painful neuropathy.

Nutritional neuropathy from a vitamin deficiency is another form of neuropathy. Nutritional neuropathy is relatively common. Thiamine deficiency can lead to hand, feet, and calf pain. You can have extreme pain just from light touch. You may have some numbness and weakness in your extremities as well.

The administration of thiamine can reduce our symptoms. Severe nutritional deficiency can cause you to develop significant pain related to your nutritional neuropathy. If you don't get enough thiamine, you can develop beriberi. This is a result of a deficiency of vitamin B1 (thiamine).

Beriberi is a nutritional neuropathy that is widespread in rice-eating countries. It is noted in individuals who eat polished rice from which the thiamine-rich seed coat is removed.

Two types of beriberi exist. One form is called wet beriberi. In this type of beriberi, there is an accumulation of tissue fluid in your body. With dry beriberi, there are signs of starvation. If you starve yourself, you will become too thin and may become sick.

Your nervous system can degenerate if you are not obtaining a proper amount of thiamine. Also, nutritional deficiencies in a woman at the time of conception can cause abnormalities in a fetus, which can cause significant harm. Pellagra is a neuropathy caused by a nutritional deficiency. Weakness, tingling, and even pain characterize it. This neuropathy is caused by a niacin deficiency.

Niacin is also a B vitamin. Pellagra is a result of a poor diet that does not have enough niacin or doesn't have sufficient tryptophane. Tryptophan is an amino acid from which niacin can be synthesized in your body. Pellagra is more common in corn-eating communities.

Chemicals you may be exposed to can cause a neuropathy as well. Cisplatin is an agent used in chemotherapy to treat tumors. This chemical can cause you to develop a painful peripheral neuropathy as well. The neuropathy associated with this drug can cause severe pain in your extremities. However, this neuropathy is reversible at the end of your chemotherapy.

Arsenic is another chemical associated with a painful neuropathy. It can also cause renal failure. Arsenic can be toxic to your heart and can cause your heart to stop. It takes one to two weeks for you to develop a neuropathy associated with arsenic ingestion. You will have burning pain as well as tingling and numbness in your extremities associated with this neuropathy. If you have a severe neuropathy from arsenic poisoning, you may not have a good prognosis on your recovery.

Thallium is an insecticide as well as a rodentcide (kills rats and mice). It can also be used to image your heart by your cardiologist when examining you for heart disease. If you suffer from thallium poisoning, you can have pain in your abdomen as well as nausea and vomiting. Your symptoms can progress through a stoppage of your heart. You can develop a psychosis as well as confusion, which can lead to a coma.

You can develop a neuropathy within 48 hours of adjusting to this chemical. You can develop pain in both your arms and legs. In severe cases, the nerves coming off of your brain called cranial nerves can be affected as well. This chemical can affect your nerves that are involved in your breathing. If you recover from this poisoning, your recovery may never be complete. One of the hallmarks of this disease is loss of hair.

There are many causes of neuropathy. An accurate diagnosis in some instances may be hard to achieve. Sometimes, it takes many tests and multiple physicians to make your diagnosis. You will likely require an EMG/NCV for an accurate diagnosis. You should be patient with your doctor if you do not have an immediate diagnosis of your neuropathic pain.

Given that no two people are alike, if you are taking any medications and begin to take nutritional supplements you should be aware that potential drug-nutrient interactions may occur and are encouraged to consult a health care professional before using any natural product.

Combining certain prescription drugs and dietary supplements can lead to undesirable effects such as: diminished prescription drug effectiveness, reduced supplement effectiveness and impaired drug and/or supplement absorption.

Low biologically available quantities of carotenoids and riboflavin from low dietary intakes and depletion through smoking would be the main precipitating factors of Epidemic Neuropathy.[1] Omega-3 fatty acids may be an efficient neuroprotective agent for prophylaxis against peripheral neuropathy.[2]

A previous study stressed the importance of checking copper levels in addition to the "more routine" vitamin levels, such as B1, B6, B12, E, and serum folate in patients with suspected nutritional optic neuropathy after bariatric surgery.[3]

Alcoholic neuropathy can be caused by direct toxic effect of ethanol or its metabolites. However, the features of alcoholic neuropathy is influenced by concomitant thiamine-deficiency state, having so far caused the obscure clinical pathological entity of alcoholic neuropathy.[4] Chronic magnesium depletion has also been linked to polyneuropathy.[5] Fish oil might be useful as an adjuvant therapy for the prevention and treatment of diabetic neuropathies.[6]

Vitamin D insufficiency is associated with self-reported peripheral neuropathy symptoms as well.[7]

References

1.      Barnouin J, Perez Cristia R, Chassagne M, et al. Vitamin and nutritional status in Cuban smokers and nonsmokers in the context of an emerging epidemic neuropathy. Int J Vitam Nutr Res. 2000;70(3):126-138.

2.      Ghoreishi Z, Esfahani A, Djazayeri A, et al. Omega-3 fatty acids are protective against paclitaxel-induced peripheral neuropathy: a randomized double-blind placebo controlled trial. BMC Cancer. 2012;12:355.

3.      Rapoport Y, Lavin PJ. Nutritional Optic Neuropathy Caused by Copper Deficiency After Bariatric Surgery. J Neuroophthalmol. 2016;36(2):178-181.

4.      Hattori N, Koike H, Sobue G. [Metabolic and nutritional neuropathy]. Rinsho Shinkeigaku. 2008;48(11):1026-1027.

5.      De Leeuw I, Engelen W, De Block C, Van Gaal L. Long term magnesium supplementation influences favourably the natural evolution of neuropathy in Mg-depleted type 1 diabetic patients (T1dm). Magnes Res. 2004;17(2):109-114.

6.      Li MY, Wang YY, Cao R, et al. Dietary fish oil inhibits mechanical allodynia and thermal hyperalgesia in diabetic rats by blocking nuclear factor-kappaB-mediated inflammatory pathways. J Nutr Biochem. 2015;26(11):1147-1155.

7.      Soderstrom LH, Johnson SP, Diaz VA, Mainous AG, 3rd. Association between vitamin D and diabetic neuropathy in a nationally representative sample: results from 2001-2004 NHANES. Diabet Med. 2012;29(1):50-55.

# 26. OSTEOPOROSIS

If you suffer from osteoporosis, you will have a progressive reduction in the density of your bones. The normal composition of your bones is preserved. Osteoporosis affects 20 million Americans and results in more than 1.3 million bone fractures in the United States every year. In a lifetime, women lose more than half of their spongy bone, which comprises the center of bones, and approximately 30 percent of the nonspongy (compact) bone, which composes the outer aspect of these bones.

Approximately 30 percent of all postmenopausal Caucasian women will suffer from fractures related to osteoporosis. More than one third of all women and one sixth of all men over 65 years of age will sustain a hip fracture.

During your lifetime, bone is constantly being made and is constantly being lost. In normal circumstances, the production and reduction of your bone is balanced. Osteoporosis can result if you do not make enough bone or if you have an accelerated decrease in your bone minerals and the matrix structure (the components of your bone which make your bones hard) of your bone or both.

Genetics can affect differences in bone density and these differences are the result of a gene that is linked to your vitamin D receptor gene. Variations of the vitamin D receptor gene result in differences in bone density changes of 10 percent to 12 percent in osteoporosis-prone individuals. Your bone density will continue to increase throughout your life until you reach an age where your bone density becomes stable.

When you approach 40, your bone density can begin to decline. Bone density decreases are noted in women before menopause. In men, a decrease in their bone density occurs somewhere between 20 to 40 years of age. In women, after menopause has occurred, the rate of bone loss accelerates.

Osteoporosis is usually diagnosed when a fracture occurs. Fractures may occur in your vertebra (compression fracture). However, your wrists, hips, ribs, pelvic bone, and your leg bones can sustain fractures. The bones in your spine can have a loss of height, which is called a compression fracture. If you have osteoporosis, your bones become more porous. This means that the bones in your body develop holes, which in turn weaken the structure of your bones.

All of your bones can be affected, and each of your bones can be at an increased risk for a fracture. If you have a low calcium intake and are not physically active, you are also at risk of developing osteoporosis.

Hyperthyroidism and hyperparathyroidism in addition to excessive cortisone (a steroid) may be causes of osteoporosis. It is important for your body to absorb calcium through your gastrointestinal system. If you have a history of a gastrectomy (removal of a portion of your stomach), cirrhosis of the liver, or any other gastrointestinal malabsorption syndrome, you are more prone to develop osteoporosis.

If you have a history of multiple myeloma or leukemia, you may develop osteoporosis. The exact cause of this finding is presently unknown. Alcohol can contribute to your development of osteoporosis. Chemotherapy can also cause osteoporosis. Steroid use has been implicated as a cause of osteoporosis as well. A plain X-ray cannot make a diagnosis of osteoporosis. You will need a DEXA test for a true diagnosis.

Osteoporosis can cause your vertebra to compress. This is called a compression fracture. Essentially your vertebra collapses. This disease can be very painful. If you have a vertebral compression in your mid back, for example, there will usually be a decrease in the height of your affected (compressed) bone that can be seen on X-ray. Sometimes a bone scan is needed to diagnosis osteoporosis. If you have a bone scan, a doctor will inject a radioactive material into your vein. You will have a picture of your body taken by a special camera.

Compression fractures, which were not diagnosed by other means, can be detected by a bone scan. Osteoporosis can also be diagnosed by measuring your bone mineral density. Your bone density value will be compared to a normal value that is noted for young adults of your same sex. A bone density test can predict the probability of you developing a fracture related to your bone density value.

Quantitative computed tomography can also be used and is effective for diagnosing osteoporosis because it will not only measure your bone mineral density, but this test can also measure the density of your spongy bone within your back and hip bones. However, this test is expensive and will expose you to radiation.

ifferent types of tests are being used and being developed to diagnosis osteoporosis. Bone scanning can be useful for the diagnosis of compression fractures. If you have a decreased bone density, your doctor should attempt to determine the cause of your osteoporosis.

Sometimes your doctor needs to obtain blood samples from you for further testing. Your doctor may take some blood from you to be sent to a lab to measure the calcium, organic phosphate, and alkaline phosphatase in your bloodstream. These minerals are usually normal if you have osteoporosis. However, your alkaline phosphate may be higher if you have a fracture. Vitamin D can help you increase your calcium absorption through your gastrointestinal tract by up to 65 percent.

Smoking on the other hand, increases the rate of bone loss. Hip and spinal bone fractures are higher in men and women who smoke. Nicotine can inhibit absorption of calcium that is needed for bone health. Osteoporosis in men can be diagnosis by a bone mass measurement. This is a special type of x-ray that emits a trace amount of radiation. Middle-aged men who have complaints of back or hip pain may be candidates for a bone mass measurement as well as a measurement of the testosterone in their bloodstream. You should avoid steroid injections.

As previously stated, the absorption of calcium from your gastrointestinal system decreases with age. The United Stated recommended dietary allowance of calcium is up to 1,000 milligrams per day. Calcium can retard your osteoporosis but cannot completely stop it. An increase in calcium in your bloodstream may not protect you from compression fractures of the bones in your spine.

Calcium therapy can help you if you are a woman and postmenopausal. Some endocrinologists have recommended that if you are postmenopausal that you should consume 1,500 milligrams per day of calcium.

Calcitonin is another drug that you could possibly take to prevent bone loss in your vertebral bodies throughout your spine. Calcitonin is most effective in early and late menopause. Calcitonin is available for intranasal use. Calcitonin has been shown to produce pain-relieving effects. Calcitonin is most useful if you have a history of osteoporosis and have chronic pain related to fractures related to your osteoporosis.

If you have had a fracture of one of the bones in your spine, treament that puts bone cement into your bone can be used to treat any compression fracture that you may have. The techniques that use this cement are called vertebroplasty and kyphoplasty.

Vertebroplasty involves the injection of bone cement into your vertebral bones. Kyphyplasty introduces a surgical instrument into one of the bones in your spine with intent to elevate the compressed bone. When this instrument is withdrawn, the space left is filled with bone cement. Each of these procedures remains to be studied.

Bisphosphonates are an important class of drug for the treatment of osteoporosis. These drugs can increase the minerals in the bones throughout your body. Furthermore, the chance of you having a vertebral fracture is decreased if you are in late menopause. Examples of these drugs include etidronate and alendronate. Further research is being done with respect to these drugs in the prevention of bone fractures.

However, these drugs will not reverse osteoporosis. There are other drugs available for women who have osteoporosis. Fosamax and Actonel are two of the drugs commonly used to decrease the progression of osteoporosis. Fosamax slows the cycle of bone breakdown. If the rate of bone breakdown is decreased, there is a reduced chance of you having a fracture.

Given that no two people are alike, if you are taking any medications and begin to take nutritional supplements you should be aware that potential drug-nutrient interactions may occur and are encouraged to consult a health care professional before using any natural product. Combining certain prescription drugs and dietary supplements can lead to undesirable effects such as: diminished prescription drug effectiveness, reduced supplement effectiveness and impaired drug and/or supplement absorption.

The prevalence of vitamin D, insufficiency is high. Vitamin D in the food supply is limited and most often inadequate to prevent deficiencies. Supplemental vitamin D is likely necessary to avoid deficiency, especially in winter months. Most cells and tissues in the human body have vitamin D receptors that stimulate the nuclear transcription of various genes to alter cellular function. Vitamin D, appears to have an effect on numerous disease states and disorders, including osteoporosis.[1]

Tridax procumbens flavonoids could be a potential anabolic agent to treat patients with bone loss-associated diseases such as osteoporosis.[2] Vitamin D(3) (cholecalciferol) sufficiency is essential for maximizing bone health. Vitamin D enhances intestinal absorption of calcium and phosphorus. sun exposure or ingesting at least 800-1000 IU of vitamin D(3) daily. Patients being treated for osteoporosis should be adequately supplemented with calcium and vitamin D to maximize the benefit of treatment.[3,4]

Fortification of bread and cereals is a feasible way to improve vitamin D nutrition in elderly nursing home residents.[5] The diet of a large part of society is not properly balanced which can cause abnormalities in achieving proper bone mineralization. Long-term deficiencies in calcium and vitamin D in daily diet are the cause for taking dietary supplements. Unfortunately, some preparations on the market do not have adequate storage. It happens that these preparations are poorly absorbed and the amount of active compound is too low.[6]

Onion juice consumption showed a positive modulatory effect on the bone loss and bone mineral density by improving antioxidant activities and thus can be recommended for treating various bone-related disorders, especially osteoporosis.[7] Furthermore, coffee consumption may have protective benefits on bone health in Korean postmenopausal women in moderate amounts.[8]

References

1.      Grober U. [Vitamin D--an old vitamin in a new perspective]. Med Monatsschr Pharm. 2010;33(10):376-383.

2.      Al Mamun MA, Hosen MJ, Islam K, Khatun A, Alam MM, Al-Bari MA. Tridax procumbens flavonoids promote osteoblast differentiation and bone formation. Biol Res. 2015;48:65.

3.      Holick MF. Optimal vitamin D status for the prevention and treatment of osteoporosis. Drugs Aging. 2007;24(12):1017-1029.

4.      Bendik I, Friedel A, Roos FF, Weber P, Eggersdorfer M. Vitamin D: a critical and essential micronutrient for human health. Front Physiol. 2014;5:248.

5.      Costan AR, Vulpoi C, Mocanu V. Vitamin D fortified bread improves pain and physical function domains of quality of life in nursing home residents. J Med Food. 2014;17(5):625-631.

6.      Kostecka M. The role of healthy diet in the prevention of osteoporosis in perimenopausal period. Pak J Med Sci. 2014;30(4):763-768.

7.      Law YY, Chiu HF, Lee HH, Shen YC, Venkatakrishnan K, Wang CK. Consumption of onion juice modulates oxidative stress and attenuates the risk of bone disorders in middle-aged and post-menopausal healthy subjects. Food Funct. 2016;7(2):902-912.

8.      Choi E, Choi KH, Park SM, Shin D, Joh HK, Cho E. The Benefit of Bone Health by Drinking Coffee among Korean Postmenopausal Women: A Cross-Sectional Analysis of the Fourth & Fifth Korea National Health and Nutrition Examination Surveys. PLoS One. 2016;11(1):e0147762.

Arthritis is a degeneration of your joints that causes you to experience joint pain. Arthritis can be caused wear and tear of your joints (osteoarthritis) or from inflammation of your joints (rheumatoid arthritis). Approximately one out of seven people has some form of arthritis, and there are many different types. More than 35 million people in the United States suffer from this disease, and every year the treatment costs the United States billions of dollars.

Inflammation that occurs in your joints can cause you to have pain as well as swelling of your joints. Cartilage is a tough, slippery layer of tissue that covers the surfaces where bones contact each other in joints. In degenerative arthritis, the cartilages in your joints wear out. A joint liner called a synovium lines the inside of your joints. The synovium contains a multitude of pain fibers. When the synovium swells, it causes release of pain signals in the area where the swelling occurs.

Approximately 25 percent of people with arthritis are unable to carry out their normal activities of daily living. This means that they have difficulty shopping, driving, and dressing. If you suffer from arthritis, your pain may come and go. More than 50 percent of people with arthritis however, report that they have pain that is constant. If you have osteoarthritis arthritis, you will experience stiffness of your joints in the morning but that the stiffness progressively decreases as you become more active.

With rheumatoid arthritis, your pain will be constant. If you have the onset of joint pain that involves one joint such as the joint in your great toe, this usually signifies gout. If you have a relative who has a history of rheumatoid arthritis, you run the risk of developing this type of arthritis. If you have had weight loss as well as chronic fatigue, you must include this in your pain diary. Weight loss and fatigue can be associated with rheumatoid arthritis.

Your doctor may use a needle and syringe to extract fluid from your joints. Your doctor will look at the fluid to see whether it is clear. Normal joint fluid should be clear. If you have osteoarthritis, the fluid can be straw colored. Other types of arthritis that you may have include rheumatoid arthritis or gout. Your fluid may be yellow. Your doctor will examine your fluids for cells. Your doctor also will obtain blood from you. Your blood will be examined for any elevation in your white cells (a sign of inflammation) and a test for rheumatoid arthritis can be done at the same time.

Your doctor may also order x rays or even a CAT scan or MRI of your painful area. Furthermore, it is not unusual for your doctor to eventually order a bone scan if your pain persists in spite of conservative treatment. A bone scan consists of injecting a very small and harmless dose of radioactive dye into your vein. After this has been done, a special camera arthritis takes a picture. If you have arthritis, there can be an increased uptake of the dye material into your painful joint, showing that the joint is inflamed.

Osteoarthritis is the most common arthritic disease. It also is called degenerative arthritis joint disease. Most of us will eventually develop osteoarthritis as we experience wear and tear of our joints. Osteoarthritis occurs when your cartilage is worn down and damaged by overuse, sometimes allowing the rigid and brittle bone ends to come into direct contact with each other.

Your bones can wear out and develop irregular growths called osteophytes that can interfere with the proper movement of your joint and cause pain. Your joints provide you with range of motion and do support your body as well. To have normal range of motion, you must have cartilage between your bones. This is why you have difficulty moving when your cartilage wears out. Osteoarthritis progresses with age. Osteoarthritis can cause not only pain in your arms and legs, but also in your spine.

Osteoarthritis can affect the elastic cartilage in your discs between your bones. These discs between your vertebral bodies in your back act as cushions between each vertebra. You also have joints in the posterior aspect of your vertebra where each joint stacks on top of one another. These joints are called facet joints. These joints can degenerate which will cause you to become stiff and will decrease your range of motion. Osteoarthritis can occur in your neck, lower back, or n your mid back.

Degenerative arthritis can affect your hips and knees as well. Your knees may become warm as well as swollen. Osteoarthritis also can affect the joints in your hands. You may notice a bony growth about the joints in your fingers. Joint pain associated with osteoarthritis usually begins gradually and progresses slowly over years. Initially, you may have degenerative arthritis but not experience pain. With the passage of time, symptoms may begin. You may notice an increase in your pain when the weather becomes cold or rains. Your pain may become severe to the point that it keeps you up at night. Osteoarthritis usually occurs in older people.

Approximately 85 percent of people over 65 develop osteoarthritis. However, only half of these people experience any symptoms. Obesity puts increased pressure and stress on your joints in your legs. Obesity is an abnormal increase in your body fat resulting in excessive weight. Obesity is measured by your body mass index (BMI). There must be a 20 percent weight gain greater than the ideal for your height and body build. If you are obese, you have an increased chance of developing osteoarthritis. Any excess weight that you carry may cause arthritis of the joints in your hips and knees.

Nonsteroidal anti-inflammatory medications are commonly used to treat osteoarthritis (for example, Celebrex, Mobic, etc.). Steroids injections into your joints can also decrease the inflammation of your knee joints, which will decrease your pain. Your doctor can also inject hyaluronic acid into your joints for pain modification. Glucosamine, which is available without a prescription, has been demonstrated to decrease pain associated with osteoarthritis. If you persist with chronic pain and disability, consultation with an orthopedic surgeon may be indicated to see if you would benefit from a total joint replacement.

Rheumatic arthritis is characterized by redness, warmth, swelling, and painful joints. If you have rheumatoid arthritis, you will have decreased range of motion of some of your joints in your body. You also may complain of stiffness. This disease attacks the synovial linings of your joints as well as the tendons about your joints.

If you develop rheumatoid arthritis, you may suffer weakness and weight loss. The exact cause of rheumatoid arthritis is un-known, but approximately 43 million people in the United States suffer from rheumatoid arthritis. Rheumatoid arthritis affects men and women, all rheumatoid arthritisces, and all ages. Family history plays an important role in the development of rheumatoid arthritis.

Rheumatoid arthritis may result from an abnormality in your immune system. Your antibodies may attack your joints to cause significant arthritis within your joints. It can usually have a slow onset. However, be aware that it can have an acute rheumatoid arthritis onset as well. The onset of rheumatoid arthritis occurs more often in the winter.

You probably have rheumatoid arthritis if you have four of the following seven criteria: 1.morning stiffness around your joints, 2.arthritis of three or more joints, 3.arthritis of your hands, 4.arthritis that occurs on both sides of your body, 5.boney nodules over your bony joints, 6.an elevated rheumatoid factor in your bloodstream, 7.X-ray determination of your joints.

The treatment of rheumatoid arthritis is to relieve your pain, preserve joint rheumatoid range of motion and decrease your joint inflammation. In addition, your doctor will want to maintain as much range of motion about your joints as possible. Splinting, exercises and strengthening exercises can be extremely beneficial to you. Occasionally, you may need a brace on one of your extremities.

Usually nonsteroidal anti-inflammatory drugs are prescribed for the management of your arthritic pain. As mentioned with regard to osteoarthritis-tis, the COX-2 inhibitors are safer for your gastrointestinal system than the older nonsteroidal anti-inflammatory drugs. Some doctors prescribe medications such as gold compounds, antimalarials, and sulfasalazine. However, each of these drugs has the potential to cause serious side effects. Steroids also may be necessary to decrease the inflammation of your joints. Steroids typically decrease pain and swelling in your joints and can be very effective.

If these methods do not relieve your pain, you may be a candidate for immunosuppressive therapy. Immunosuppressive therapy is the administration of a drug that eliminates or lessens an immune response. Methotrexate is used frequently for the treatment of your rheumatoid arthritis.

Methotrexate can cause liver pathology. Surgery is the last resort for the treatment of rheumatoid arthritis and consists of total joint replacement. If your pain becomes intolerable and if you have significant limitations in joint function, surgery can provide you with relief. Joint replacements are now available for hips, knees, shoulders, elbows, and ankles.

Disease-modifying antirheumatic drugs (DMARDs) can substantially reduce the inflammation of rheumatoid arthritis. DMARDs can reduce or prevent joint damage, preserve joint structure and function, and enable a person to continue his or her daily activities. Drugs in this class include hydroxychloroquine (Plaquenil), methotrexate (Rheuma-trex), gold salts (Ridaurheumatoid arthritis, Solganal), D-penicillamine (Depen, Cuprimine), sulfasalazine (Azulfidine®, azathioprine (Imurheumatoid arthritisn), leflunomide (Arheumatoid arthritisva), and cyclosporine (Sandimmune, Neorheumatoid arthritisl).Severheumatoid arthritisl weeks to months of treatment are often necessary before the effects of DMARDs become evident.

Ankylosing spondylitis is an inflammatory disease that predominantly affects men. Pain usually begins in the back and sacroiliac joint (the joint where the back and hip bones meet) early in life. An x-rheumatoid arthritisy of the spine of a male with ankylosing spondylitis appears as bamboo and is called a bamboo spine. This pattern is also seen on MRI imaging studies.

Ankylosing spondylitis usually affects men before the age of 40. If you have ankylosing spondylitis, you may develop arthritis of your spine as well as the large joints in your body. Ankylosing spondylitis is present in 8 percent of Caucasians and 3 percent of African American men. A marker in the bloodstream called HLA-B27 is present in 90 percent of patients who have ankylosing spondylitis. Ankylosing spondylitis has been observed in rheumatoid arthritists when the HLA-B27 gene is expressed.

Usually ankylosing spondylitis will become manifest in a male around age 20. This arthritic disease does occur in women, but the symptoms are more prominent in men. If you do suffer from ankylosing spondylitis-tis, your primary symptoms may be pain in your hip joints. You may have progressive decrease of your back range of motion. You may have some pain in the joints of your arms and legs as well. X-rays have shown arthritis in sacroiliac joints. Over time, your spine will continue to stiffen. The onset of ankylosing spondylitis is gradual. You have a normal curve in your lower back that will become straight. You may have difficulty expanding your chest to take a breath.

If your ankylosing spondylitis worsens, your entire spine may become fused, which restricts your motion about your spine in all directions. The earliest x-ray changes usually occur in your sacroiliac joints. Erosion of these joints becomes evident. The outer rings of your discs in your spine become calcified.

Furthermore, calcification of the vertical ligaments that run in front and back of your vertebral bones occur. When this happens, if you have an x-rheumatoid arthritisy of your spine, it will appear as a bamboo stick. Remember that rheumatoid arthritis affects mostly small joints. Ankylosing spondylitis affects large joints. Osteoarthritis does not usually affect your sacroiliac joints.

If you have ankylosing spondylitis, physical therapy and nonsteroidal anti-inflammatory drugs are important for the treatment of the pain associated with this disease. No treatment is currently available that will eradicate ankylosing spondylitis. Occasionally stronger analgesics such as opioids are needed to control your pain.

Sulfasalazine is sometimes useful for pain for arthritis in your arms and legs. The problem with ankylosing spondylitis is that you can have pain that is severe over decades of your life. The severity of the pain associated with this disease varies greatly. Approximately 10 percent of patients have disability so severe that they are unable to return to work after 10 years.

Gout is one of the most painful arthritic diseases. Gout results from the formation crystals of uric acid that are deposited into joint spaces between your bones. These uric acid crystals deposited into your joints cause inflammation with swelling, redness, and warmth about your joint. Gouty arthritis comprises 5 percent of all cases of arthritis. We all have the formation of uric acid in our bodies.

Uric acid is formed in your body from the breakdown of chemicals called purines that are found in many foods. You should avoid foods that will elevate your uric acid blood level. If you have a history of gout, avoid excessive meat and seafood in your diet. Do not eat gravy. Avoid yeast products, including beer and other alcoholic beverages. You must also avoid oatmeal, asparagus, cauliflower, and mushrooms.

Uric acid is dissolved in your bloodstream and is excreted through the kidneys. If your kidneys do not eliminate enough uric acid from your bloodstream, the uric acid will increase in your bloodstream. If you eat a lot of liver, beans, or peas, you may increase the uric acid in your bloodstream. If the uric acid forms crystals and deposits these crystals into your joints, gout will develop.

In many people, the uric acid deposits affect the joints in their great toes. The big toe is affected in approximately 75 percent of people suffering gout. The ankles, heels, knees, wrists, and fingers may also be affected by gouty arthritis.

If you have a family history of gouty arthritis, you run the risk of developing this disease. Gout is more common in men than in women and is more common in adults than in children. Obesity increases the risk of developing gout. An excess consumption of alcohol also interferes with the excretion of uric acid from your body.

The increased uric acid that occurs from excessive alcohol consumption can form crystals and deposit these crystals into your joints. Adult men between the ages of 40 and 50 are most likely to develop gout. Gout is occasionally seen in women. It occurs before menopause. For some reason, people who have had organ transplants are more susceptible to gout.

A diagnosis of gout can be made by with fluid analysis from your painful joints and analyzing the fluid for uric acid. When your gout attack is severe, you may be totally incapacitated. If your gout is not treated, you may develop severe pathology of your affected joints. The prevalence of gout for men is approximately 14 cases per 1,000 men, whereas the prevalence in women is approximately 6 cases per 1,000 women. Estrogen hormones noted in women can help the body eliminate uric acid. For this reason, gout is rarely seen in premenopausal women.

When a gout attack occurs, the maximum pain associated with the gout usually occurs in approximately the first 10 hours. In general, attacks resolve in less than 14 days. Uric acid crystals can not only be deposited in your joints, they can also form in your soft tissues. A collection of uric acid crystals in your tissues can form a lump (called a tophi), often noted on the outer edges of your forearms.

Be aware that if you have gout, you have an increased risk of developing kidney stones. These stones are usually composed of uric acid. If you have gout, you also have a higher risk of developing a kidney disease. Finding uric acid crystals in the fluid of your joints makes the diagnosis of gout.

Uric acid crystals are usually formed when your uric acid level exceeds 6.8 mg/dL. Sometimes overproduction of uric acid is related to a genetic disorder. Excessive exercise can also increase uric acid, as can obesity. Starvation or dehydration can increase uric acid. Thyroid disease can also increase uric acid. Diuretics (medications that make you urinate, such as furosemide (Lasix) and hydrochlorothiazide (HCTZ), a common blood pressure medicine) and cyclosporine A (an immunosuppressive medicine) can increase the uric acid concentration in the bloodstream.

The initial treatment of gout may include nonsteroidal anti-inflammatory medications or steroids or colchicine. The use of COX-2 inhibitors is under investigation. Steroids can be used to treat gout and can be given orally or by injection into your muscle.

Given that no two people are alike, if you are taking any medications and begin to take nutritional supplements you should be aware that potential drug-nutrient interactions may occur and are encouraged to consult a health care professional before using any natural product. Combining certain prescription drugs and dietary supplements can lead to undesirable effects such as: diminished prescription drug effectiveness, reduced supplement effectiveness and impaired drug and/or supplement absorption.

The aim of the first global systematic review on selected nutrition pharmaceuticals was to synthesize and evaluate scientific relevant data available in the literature for nutritional effects on osteoarthritis. Evidences that can support health, physiological or functional benefit on osteoarthritis (Vitamin D showed a pro-catabolic effect in vitro and the polyphenol, Genistein, had only anti-inflammatory potency. The evaluation of the clinical data showed that avocado/soybean unsaponifiables  were the studied ingredients to present a good evidence of efficacy for osteoarthritis treatment.[1]

The effects of a rheumatoid arthritis administered combination of a glucosamine-chondroitin-quercetin glucoside supplement on the synovial fluid properties of patients with osteoarthritis and rheumatoid arthritis were investigated . A large dose of vitamin B(6) supplementation (100 mg/day) suppressed pro-inflammatory cytokines in patients with rheumatoid arthritis in one study.[2]

Osteoarthritis showed a significant improvement in pain symptoms, daily activities (walking and climbing up and down stairs), and visual analogue scale, and changes in the synovial fluid properties with respect to the protein concentration, molecular size of hyaluronic acid, and chondroitin 6-sulphate concentrations were also observed. However, no such effects were observed in the rheumatoid arthritis patients.[3]

A pilot clinical trial showed that daily supplementation with oral hyaluronic acid from a natural extract of chicken combs (Hyal-Joint) was useful to enhance several markers of quality of life in adults with osteoarthritis of the knee. Researchers examined the effect of dietary supplementation with an extract of chicken combs with a high content of hyaluronic acid (60%) on pain noted an increased quality of life in subjects with osteoarthritis of the knee.[4]

Sesame seed is a natural and safe substance that may have beneficial effects in patients with knee OA, and it may provide new complementary and adjunctive treatment in these patients.[5] A study examined the nutritional status of Danish rheumatoid arthritis patients and addressed the question of whether or not rheumatoid arthritis can be directly influenced by dietary manipulation. Those following the diet demonstrated a significant improvement in the duration of morning stiffness, the number of swollen joints, pain status, and a reduced cost of medicine in this study.

References

1.      Henrotin Y, Lambert C, Couchourel D, Ripoll C, Chiotelli E. Nutrheumatoid arthritisceuticals: do they represent a new erheumatoid arthritisin the management of osteoarthritis? - a narrheumatoid arthritistive review from the lessons taken with five products. Osteoarthritis Cartilage. 2011;19(1):1-21.

2.      Huang SC, Wei JC, Wu DJ, Huang YC. Vitamin B(6) supplementation improves pro-inflammatory responses in patients with rheumatoid arthritis. Eur J Clin Nutr. 2010;64(9):1007-1013.

3.      Matsuno H, Nakamurheumatoid arthritisH, Katayama K, et al. Effects of an orheumatoid arthritisl administrheumatoid arthritistion of glucosamine-chondroitin-quercetin glucoside on the synovial fluid properties in patients with osteoarthritis and rheumatoid arthritis. Biosci Biotechnol Biochem. 2009;73(2):288-292.

4.      Kalman DS, Heimer M, Valdeon A, Schwartz H, Sheldon E. Effect of a naturheumatoid arthritisl extrheumatoid arthritisct of chicken combs with a high content of hyaluronic acid (Hyal-Joint) on pain relief and quality of life in subjects with knee osteoarthritis: a pilot rheumatoid arthritisndomized double-blind placebo-controlled trial. Nutr J. 2008;7:3.

5.      Khadem Haghighian M, Alipoor B, Malek Mahdavi A, Eftekhar Sadat B, Asghari Jafarheumatoid arthritisbadi M, Moghaddam A.

Effects of sesame seed supplementation on inflammatory factors and oxidative stress biomarkers in patients with knee osteoarthritis. Acta Med Irheumatoid arthritisn. 2015;53(4):207-213.

Shingles is a painful disease that is caused by the same virus (herpes zoster virus) that caused chickenpox when you were a child. This virus is rendered dormant by your immune system when your body has healed from the chicken pox infection. This same virus may affect some of the nerves that go out of your spinal cord to your chest or face. One or more nerves can be affected. Shingles occurs in those patients who have had chickenpox.

Usually the shingles pain stays on one side of your body. The shingles virus will remain in a nerve after your chickenpox has healed. This area is called your dorsal root ganglia. This virus is dormant but typically reactivates when you age. This reactivation usually occurs after your immune system has been weakened, usually by another viral infection such as the flu or common cold. If you have cancer, you may be prone to develop shingles as well.

Sometimes there is no known reason why you develop shingles. If you have had contact with an individual who has active chicken pox, there is a chance that you could develop shingles. However, this scenario is rare. You need to be aware that shingles does not increase during seasonal chicken pox outbreaks. When the virus is reactivated in your dorsal root ganglia, it goes along your nerves to your nerve endings. The virus at this time will cause your skin to develop painful skin lesions.

You need to be aware that this virus can affect any part of your central nervous system. In rare cases, this virus can even affect your brain; this is called encephalitis. The virus has been reported in some cases to affect the sympathetic ganglia as well, which can cause severe burning pain. This will cause you to have symptoms that mimic reflex sympathetic dystrophy.

Following a chicken pox infection, antibodies are made in your body to fight the chicken pox virus. This is the reason why you usually do not get chicken pox again. However, if your immune system is compromised for any reason, your body's ability to combat the virus is greatly reduced. This is the reason why you may develop shingles. If your immune system appears to be attacked, your body will immediately fight the shingles virus by producing antibodies to the virus.

After you have had the onset of shingles, you may develop postherpetic neuralgia. This is a chronic pain syndrome that occurs following the onset of shingles. When you have the onset of shingles, you will have blisters as well as burning sensations in your skin where the infected nerves run.

When you develop post-herpetic neuralgia, which can persist for years, after your skin lesions have healed.

If you are between the ages of 40 and 60, the chances of you developing post-herpetic neuralgia are 20 percent. If you are over 60 years of age, your chance of developing post-herpetic neuralgia will increase to 50 percent. Post-herpetic neuralgia is a difficult entity to treat.

Post-herpetic neuralgia can cause you to have agonizing pain as well as suffering. Some individuals have even committed suicide to escape this terrible pain. Sometimes you can develop burning pain associated with the herpes zoster virus. However, it may be some time before your skin lesions appear.

Before you develop a skin rash, the diagnosis of herpes zoster is difficult to make. After your skin lesions erupt, the diagnosis is easier to make. If you have pain in your mid chest, you may be incorrectly diagnosed with a coronary artery disease or pneumonia. If your doctor wants to confirm your diagnosis, the virus should be isolated from your pustules no later than seven days after they erupted.

Be aware that if you have severe burning pain that develops on one side of your body, you may or may not have a skin eruption but you can have shingles. Sometimes the lack of a skin eruption confuses doctors as to whether you actually have the onset of shingles, because skin lesions are so common.

If you do develop skin eruptions, the lesions will begin as redness. The redness over your skin will turn to blisters. The blisters can form pus. Eventually these lesions on your skin break down. A crust then forms. If the virus affects your skin, in addition to your nerves, you may develop scars as well as loss of skin pigment about the infected site.

Be aware that the virus can travel to your eyes. If you or anyone in your family has developed shingles and begins to complain of eye pain, this is a medical emergency. You must contact an ophthalmologist immediately. If left untreated, the virus may blind you.

Shingles may be preceded by other events. Be aware that psychological stress can also trigger the onset of shingles. If you have a history of a prolonged use of steroids, you may also be prone to develop shingles.

For reasons yet unknown, the Caucasian race appears to have a higher incidence of shingles than other races. Your chest will be most affected by shingles.

A nerve coming off of your brain that distributes branches to your face called the trigeminal nerve is the next most common nerve affected. Next the nerves off of your neck (called the cranial nerves) are affected, followed by the nerves coming off of your spinal cord that go to your legs (called the lumbar nerves). As you can see, shingles can affect nerves all over your body.

After you have been diagnosed with shingles, your doctor will probably treat you with an antiviral drug.. Acyclovir, famciclovir, and valacyclovir can be used for the treatment of your viral infection. Antiviral medications are used to decrease the intensity and duration of your shingles and are used to prevent the chronic pain associated with post-herpetic neuralgia.

Be aware that you can still have the onset of post-herpetic neuralgia even after treatment with these antiviral agents. Pain associated with post-herpetic neuralgia can be described as aching, burning, or stabbing.

The worst pain is pain that is triggered by light touch such as clothing, bathing, or lying on a mattress. Sometimes cold weather or cold water can worsen your pain. Post-herpetic neuralgia is a dreaded complication of shingles.

If you develop shingles and if your pain lasts longer than six weeks after your skin lesions have disappeared, you may have developed post-herpetic neuralgia. Be aware that a certain proportion of individuals who develop post-herpetic neuralgia will improve over time with no treatment.

f you have post-herpetic neuralgia, the chances are that you will have im-proved by 12 months. Approximately 30 percent of individuals who develop post-herpetic neuralgia still complain of pain after one year. Two percent of individuals who suffer from post-herpetic neuralgia will have pain longer than five years.

Doctors of different specialties treat shingles. Your primary care doctor or a dermatologist may treat you. You may have to go to an emergency room because of severe pain and be treated by that doctor. You may also be referred to a pain-medicine specialist. Psychologists are also valuable in the management of your pain. All of these health-care providers can significantly help you manage your pain. You may find that each of these providers uses a different modality for the treatment of your pain. If your pain is moderate, a mild analgesic such as Ultracet (tramadol) or a mild narcotic such as

Darvocet or Tylenol with codeine may suffice for the management of your pain. If your pain becomes excruciating, these medications will not provide you with any significant pain relief. At this time, you may require more potent opioid medication such as Percocet or Vicodin.

If these stronger narcotic drugs do not provide you with relief, you may require the administration of a strong opioid medication such as morphine. If you develop post-herpetic neuralgia, avoid stressful situations that may worsen your pain. Avoid situations that cause you significant anxiety and/or depression. If you live in a cold environment, dress warmly.

In addition to antiviral agents, your doctor may prescribe steroids. Lotions, different types of patches, nonsteroidal anti-inflammatory drugs, antidepressants, and muscle relaxants may all be needed to control your pain. You may even need injections of numbing medicines into your nerves. Placement of local anesthetics around your sympathetic nerves may be of benefit in reducing your pain, especially if the injection is done soon after the onset of your pain.

Topical agents are frequently used to treat shingles pain. These agents accelerate the healing of your skin and can decrease the pain associated with the shingles virus. However, topical anesthetics administered at the time that you develop shingles will not affect the development of post-herpetic neuralgia. Compresses or Burrow's solution or calamine lotion placed directly over your painful site can decrease the pain associated with acute herpes zoster.

A patch has been developed for the treatment of shingles. This patch called the Lidoderm patch has proven to be extremely useful in the management of shingles and post-herpetic neuralgia pain. A local anesthetic called lidocaine is placed within a patch system.

The lidocaine is placed within an adhesive. The adhesive binds to your skin. Another type of transdermal (skin) drug-delivery system is a clonidine transdermal patch. This is placed over the area of your maximal pain. This drug is a drug that controls an individual's blood pressure.

Tricyclic antidepressants are frequently used for the management of pain associated with post-herpetic neuralgia. In fact, tricyclic antidepressants are used to treat a variety of chronic pain syndromes.

The exact mechanism by which these drugs decrease your pain is unknown. If narcotics are to be used, mild narcotics should be initiated, as previously stated. Propoxyphene (Darvon) has been successfully used in a geriatric population for a several week duration. Morphine is commonly used for severe pain. Baclofen, Amantadine, and Elavil can decrease your burning pain associated with post-herpetic neuralgia while anticonvulsant medications can lessen your sharp, shooting pain.

Another topical drug that is sometimes used is capsaicin cream. It can be purchased over the counter and can also be purchased by prescription at a higher concentration. A newer anticonvulsant drug called Lyrica (pregabilin) is very effective in decreasing your pain.

Shingles pain may be decreased by physical therapy. Heat, cold, and massage are frequently used for the management of your pain. Some-times a transcutaneous electrical nerve stimulator (TENS) can be helpful. The TENS unit, however, is not frequently prescribed because on occasion it could worsen the pain associated with shingles. Water therapy can be helpful because the warm water can be soothing and may also desensitize the nerves that are causing the severe pain.

If your activities of daily living are limited because of your pain, consult an occupational therapist to learn how to preserve your daily-living activities. Sometimes your doctor may want to put numbing medicine mixed with a steroid around your affected nerve. If you are experiencing pain in your chest wall, for example, your doctor may place an injection into the nerve that provides sensation to your chest. This nerve is called the intercostal nerve.

The type of nerve block used to treat your pain depends on the type of pain that you have. The pain associated with post-herpetic neuralgia can be somatic, sympathetic, or central. The somatic pain follows a certain nerve that is affected. Sympathetic pain can decrease the blood flow to your tissues and causes you to have a burning pain.

Central pain is a result of rewiring of your central nervous system. For this type of pain, you need a different type of block. Sympathetic nerve blocks, if done early, can relieve pain associated with shingles and can also decrease the incidence of developing post-herpetic neuralgia. To be effective, they should be performed within the first two months after the onset of your symptoms.

Stellate ganglion blocks are used for pain in your head, neck, and arms. Thoracic epidural blocks are used for pain in your mid back and chest wall, whereas lumbar sympathetic blocks are used for the management of post-herpetic neuralgia pain in your lower extremities. The purpose of nerve blocks is to interrupt your pain impulses and to facilitate therapy and to help you increase your daily-living activities. Nerve blocks should be used if your pain is becoming too severe and cannot be controlled by non-narcotic medications.

If you have sympathetic pain that does not respond to the previously mentioned modalities, more permanent blocks of your sympathetic nervous system can be done using a modality called radiofrequency thermocoagulation. This device provides some heat about your sympathetic nerves. This device does not burn your nerves, but the heat essentially puts your nerves out of commission.

Occasionally a dorsal column stimulator can be placed in your epidural space to manage your pain. The dorsal column stimulator is essentially an epidural catheter that has electrodes on it. The number of electrodes that are used depends on the pattern of your pain. The dorsal column stimulator is placed within your body on a trial basis.

The catheter is placed on an out-patient basis with x-ray. The end of the catheter attaches to a battery pack which can be placed under your skin. How the dorsal column stimulator actually works is debated.

It is believed that the electrical interference with ascending pathways may be the mechanism for decreasing your pain impulse transmission. The use of this device has been demonstrated to be effective for the management of post-herpetic neuralgic pain that is refractory to all other modalities.

If you do obtain adequate pain relief, the stimulator is implanted permanently surgically. For pain that persists in your arms or legs and is refractory to other treatments, a nerve stimulator can be placed in that extremity to provide you with pain relief. Chemical substances that disrupt nerves have been used since 1930 for the treatment of post-herpetic neuralgia.

Phenol is an alcohol-like drug used to disrupt your nerve impulses. It also has some local anesthetic properties. The first reported use of a neurolitic solution was in 1863 by Luton. Neurolitic blocks for chronic pain management were further developed by neurosurgeons. In 1925, Dr. Doppler used phenol for disruption of nerves.

In 1955, phenol was administered in the spinal fluid of patients to disrupt their chronic pain. Alcohol has also been used to disrupt nerve signals. However, the use of the alcohol can cause post-block pain called neuritis. Whenever neurolitic chemicals are used, the procedure must be done under X-ray guidance to know where the solution is going. Sometimes the phenol must be re-administered to provide you with a good long-term block of your nerves.

If all the previous modalities fail to provide you with relief, a narcotic pump can be placed within your body. The pump consists of a reservoir about the size of a hockey puck. A newly developed snail toxin placed in this pump may give you significant pain relief. The pump is connected to a tube that runs into the fluid that surrounds your spinal cord.

Essentially this pump gives you a drop of a narcotic drug every minute or so and is another way of controlling your pain. The drug-delivery system is refilled approximately every 45 days. Before placing this pump, your doctor will do a trial of morphine or a similar drug and compare it to a salt solution (placebo) to see whether you actually obtain pain relief from this device. A snail toxin placed in the pump may also be effective.

Histopathologically, the skin lesions of acute herpes zoster are characterized by epidermal necrotic vesicles with inflammation. Nitric oxide is generated from L-arginine by nitric oxide synthase , and immune inflamma-tion involves the activation of nitric oxide synthase in both effector cells and target cells.[1]

Given that no two people are alike, if you are taking any medications and begin to take nutritional supplements you should be aware that potential drug-nutrient interactions may occur and are encouraged to consult a health care professional before using any natural product. Combining certain prescription drugs and dietary supplements can lead to undesirable effects such as: diminished prescription drug effectiveness, reduced supplement effectiveness and impaired drug and/or supplement absorption.

Foods high in arginine include chocolate, cola, grain cereals, chicken soup, gelatin, seeds, nuts and peas. The herpes family virus's outer shell is arginine. Avoid high-arginine foods, take supplemental lysine for 10 days at the onset of a shingles episode. Nuts are high in arginine, compared to lysine. If you are prone to shingles, avoid foods that are higher in arginine than lysine.

Vitamin C inhibits viral replication, and it makes sense that this ther-apy could ease an episode of shingles. It's also been noted that patients suffering with PHN have reduced blood levels of vitamin C. High-dose vitamin B12 is a treatment for shingles as well. The amino acid L-lysine, like vitamin C, inhibits the replication of the herpes zoster virus.

The possibility exists that vitamin D might affect the course of postherpetic neuralgia. As vitamin D receptors are present in a variety of human tissues, particularly immune cells, the immunomodulatory potential of vitamin D cannot be overemphasized.[2]

References
1.      Lim YJ, Chang SE, Choi JH, et al. Expression of inducible ni-tric oxide synthase in skin lesions of acute herpes zoster. J Dermatol Sci. 2002;29(3):201-205.
2.      Chao CT, Chiang CK, Huang JW, Hung KY. Vitamin D is closely linked to the clinical courses of herpes zoster: From pathogenesis to complications. Med Hypotheses. 2015;85(4):452-457.

# 29. REFLEX SYMPATHETIC DYSTROPHY

Reflex sympathetic dystrophy (RSD) affects one or more of your arms or legs but also can affect your face following a tooth extraction. Reflex sympathetic dystrophy is now called the Complex Regional Pain Syndrome (CRPS). Reflex sympathetic dystrophy is serious, painful, and potentially disabling. Pain associated with this entity is throbbing, burning, or aching.

You can have pain just to light touch (alodynia). You can have swelling of one or more of your extremities as well as either warmth or coldness depending on the phase of your RSD and sweating also occurs on the palms of your hands or the soles of your feet.

Your hair may grow faster on the extremity with RSD at first, only to progress to loss of hair on your arm or leg. Your extremity will sweat if you have RSD. It can turn color. The nails in your affected limb can grow faster on the extremity that suffers from reflex sympathetic dystrophy.

Reflex sympathetic dystrophy usually occurs following an injury. However, a heart attack or stroke can also trigger reflex sympathetic dystrophy. It can be seen in the knee as well as in the shoulder. Reflex sympathetic dystrophy occurs in 40 percent of the cases followed an injury to a muscle or a nerve. Simple bruises or sprains can also trigger reflex sympathetic dystrophy.

Fractures accounted for 25 percent of reflex sympathetic dystrophy cases. Twenty percent of the RSD patients were postoperative on an arm or leg, whereas 12 percent occurred after a heart attack. Three percent occurred after a stroke. Approximately 37 percent of patients in the study had emoional disturbances at the time of the onset of the reflex sympathetic dystrophy.

It was once thought that reflex sympathetic dystrophy was caused by an emotional problem. Many people do not suffer from emotional problems at the time of the onset of reflex sympathetic dystrophy. Treatment usually consists of oral medications as well as injection therapy by an anesthesiologist using local anesthetics. Steroids may also be used effectively to treat RSD. If you sustained actual nerve damage, your reflex sympathetic dystrophy is called causalgia or complex regional pain syndrome II. Complex regional pain syndrome I does not have a nerve injury associated with it.

Reflex sympathetic dystrophy is a syndrome that consists of burning pain, pain to touch over the skin of the injured extremity, shiny skin, and skin that has different colors consisting of either redness or a blue cyanotic color. Blue or cyanotic discoloration usually occurs when skin or other tissues do not get enough blood and oxygen. With this disease, the pain in your extremity is out of proportion to your injury.

It was originally hypothesized that if your sympathetic nervous system became hyperactive, this hyperactivity caused of reflex sympathetic dystrophy. Your sympathetic nervous system is one component of your autonomic nervous system. The other component is called the parasympathetic nervous system. Your autonomic nervous system regulates your circulation and your breathing as well as your stomach and bladder functions. You have no control over your autonomic nervous system.

Your sympathetic nervous system sends sympathetic nerve fibers to the blood vessels in your head and neck as well as to your skin, muscles and sweat glands in your arms and legs. Your hands and feet can sweat profusely if you have reflex sympathetic dystrophy and the hair on your arms and legs can grow faster or fall out.

Your sympathetic nerve fibers can also restrict circulation in certain areas of your body. Sometimes if your doctor blocks your sympathetic nerve pathways with a numbing medicine, you can have some relief of your reflex sympathetic dystrophy.

The treatment of reflex sympathetic dystrophy includes weekly repetitive sympathetic blocks up to 5 or 6 or removal of the sympathetic nerves, either surgically or by chemicals such as phenol or by intense heat. Sympathetic blocks involve placing a local anesthetic about the bundles of nerves that exist outside of your central nervous system.

These nerve bundles that are called ganglia are in your neck as well as your lower back. The ganglion in your neck influences your arm pain- while your ganglion in your lower back influences RSD pain in your leg.

For you to be diagnosed with RSD, you should have the following: An initiating traumatic event to your body (e.g. bone fracture), an onset of spontaneous pain, excruciating pain to light touch (allodynia) as well as pain from a noxious stimulus that lasts longer than expected. Your pain must be global and not just confined to a specific area.

For example, if you have injured your hand, you may have an injury to one of the nerves in your hand. Your ulnar nerve will give you pain or numbness in your last two fingers of your hand if this nerve is affected. This is the definition of a neuritis that means inflammation of a nerve. This is not RSD. This is an example of neuralgia. RSD means that the whole hand (global) is painful and not just in the distribution of one nerve.

Other signs of reflex sympathetic dystrophy include evidence of swelling of your extremity, an increase or a decrease in your skin blood flow noted by imaging as well as alterations in the color of your skin and sweating. Cold applications to your skin can worsen your pain. Movement of your joints can also cause pain if you have RSD. You skin may be shiny. Your nails should grow faster on the side of the reflex sympathetic dystrophy. At first your hair will grow faster on the side of your reflex sympathetic dystrophy but eventually your hair pattern will decrease and you may even lose hair in this area.

Tremors or spasms may be noted on the side of your reflex sympathetic dystrophy. If you have complex regional pain syndrome, you should also have complaints of stiffness at the joints where your fingers meet your hand or where your toes meet your foot. Some physicians can over diagnose complex regional pain syndrome.

Unfortunately, some surgeons call botched surgery that they did that had a bad outcome RSD. They will make a presumptive diagnosis of RSD rather than admit that he or she caused a problem. This situation however, is rare.

RSD must be treated immediately once it has been diagnosed. If you have any of these symptoms mentioned in this chapter, notify your doctor. A three-phase bone scan can be useful in diagnosing reflex sympathetic dystrophy (figure 1). This imagery is related to the distribution of a radioactive isotope throughout the body, and a nuclear medicine doctor will examine the distribution of the radioactive isotope in the affected extremity.

The distribution of the radioactive isotope is dependent upon blood flow as well as the activity of the bone. In early RSD, you will have increased blood flow and after 3 months your blood flow will be decreased. If your three-phase bone scan is negative, this does not mean that you do not have reflex sympathetic dystrophy. A three-phase bone scan may be effective for staging the early or late forms of RSD. Magnetic resonance imaging (MRI) can also aid in the diagnosis of RSD by identifying swelling in the center of your bone. This bone marrow edema is characteristic of complex regional pain syndrome. This study is more reliable than a three-phase bone scanning or plain X-ray exams.

Figure 1. Three-phase bones scan of hands. The left hand has RSD. The uptake of isotope is much higher in the left hand.

Contact and infrared thermography have both been used for the diagnosis of reflex sympathetic dystrophy, but the problem with thermography is that it can be influenced not only by skin blood flow but also by the temperature of the room environment as well as by your muscle and your deep tissue metabolism. A new method called laser Doppler imaging has been shown to be effective for the diagnosis of complex regional pain syndrome. The laser Doppler is important because the results of this study are influenced by your skin blood flow. Your skin blood flow is under the control of your autonomic nervous system.

After you have sustained an injury to your extremity, the blood vessels to your extremity initially increase in caliber. This allows more blood flow to go to your extremity. Your hand or foot will therefore, feel warm and may appear to be red. This phase usually occurs within the first month of your injury. A three-phase bone scan at this time will demonstrate increased isotope activity in your extremity, which indicates phase 1 reflex sympathetic dystrophy.

As your RSD progresses, the blood vessels to your extremity will decrease in caliber. They go from their enlarged diameter to a normal appearing diameter. This is phase II. You will have some swelling as well at this time and global pain about your extremity and sweating of your extremity as your sympathetic nervous system becomes overactive. This phase can progress on to phase III.

During phase III, your blood vessels become extremely small and you have decreased blood flow to your hand, foot, or your affected extremity. This will cause your skin to become cold. By this time, you will notice that your skin has become shiny and that the sweating in your hand or foot may have increased. A three-phase bone scan at this time can detect a significant decrease in your blood flow to your extremity. Your treating doctor should try and prevent you from progressing through these phases by being aggressive in his or her treatment.

Be aware that on rare occasions RSD can spread into more than one extremity. If you have chronic RSD, you can have skin infections associated with persistent swelling of your skin as well as blood vessels that can spontaneously rupture. You may have a change in skin pigmentation and your fingernails or pump, which sends a narcotic into your spinal fluid, needs to be implanted to control your RSD pain.

Clonidine, which is frequently prescribed as a patch over your skin, can also be administered into your epidural space for the control of your pain as well. Baclofen or a snail toxin toenails on the affected extremity can become thick and clubbed.

The frequency of reflex sympathetic dystrophy shows a peak incidence of this entity around 50 years of age. However, you must be aware that both children and elderly individuals can develop RSD.

RSD can be refractive to treatment with sympathetic blockade. This type of RSD is called sympathetically independent pain. RSD related pain that responds to sympathetic blockade is classified as sympathetically maintained pain. Sympathetically maintained pain usually has a decrease in your pain component following a sympathetic block. The onset of reflex sympathetic dystrophy can occur at any time following a traumatic event ranging from days to months.

The exact cause of reflex sympathetic dystrophy is unknown. If you have had a nerve injury where your nerve was cut, your nerve endings will attempt to grow together. The nerve endings will sprout small nerve fibers. Sometimes as your nerves attempt to grow together, the area where they come together can be extremely painful. Where the nerve endings come together can cause an extremely painful area called a neuroma. This neuroma is sensitive to the chemicals released by your sympathetic nervous system.

Females are more vulnerable to sympathetically mediated pain than males. The chemicals that are involved that cause you to have reflex sympathetic dystrophy are potentially affected by your sex hormones. It is believed that your hormone status at the time of your trauma is important for the development of the pain associated with reflex sympathetic dystrophy.

The effects of reflex sympathetic dystrophy on the central processing in your central nervous system may be the basis for the spread of reflex sympathetic dystrophy to your other extremities. Many recommendations for the treatment of reflex sympathetic dystrophy exist. Because there are so many different treatments proposed, you should be aware that no single treatment is superior to the others. Remember that no treatment for complex regional pain syndrome is consistently successful.

It is known that early recognition and active treatment of the complex regional pain syndrome improves your outcome. For example, injections of local anesthetics about your sympathetic nervous system can alleviate your symptoms of reflex sympathetic dystrophy for weeks to months.

In some instances the relief may be permanent. These types of injections must be done early following the onset of your symptoms of reflex sympathetic dystrophy. The injections can be done in your stellate ganglion, which provides sympathetic fibers to your arms, or the injections can be done in the lumbar sympathetic ganglion, which supplies sympathetic fibers to your legs and feet.

A clonidine patch can be used to decrease your pain. This patch is usually used to treat high blood pressure. However, the patch does decrease the sympathetic nervous system chemicals that can be released if you have reflex sympathetic dystrophy. The patch is usually worn for one week before it is changed.

Steroids administered by mouth are effective for the treatment of reflex sympathetic dystrophy. Steroids will decrease inflammation caused by prostaglandins. If your pain is severe, your doctor will probably prescribe a narcotic drug for you. Depending on the severity of your pain, your doctor will prescribe a mild narcotic such as Darvocet (propoxyphene) or a stronger narcotic such as methadone.

Anticonvulsive medications can be helpful in decreasing your pain. Gabapentin (Neurontin) is frequently used now for the treatment of pain associated with your complex regional pain syndrome.

Narcotic medications administered into your spinal fluid can help decrease your pain. Sometimes a morphine (Prialt) placed in the pump may also decrease your pain. Antidepressant medications such as amitriptyline have also been shown to be effective. Amitriptyline increases certain chemicals in your central nervous system that are helpful in decreasing the amount of pain that reaches your brain.

Implantation of an electrical spinal wire attached to a battery into your epidural space can also provide you with significant pain relief. This apparatus is called a dorsal column stimulator.

Psychological intervention is also helpful; because of the severity of the pain associated with reflex sympathetic dystrophy, you can develop fear, anxiety, and depression. Psychological intervention including the use of biofeedback and sometimes hypnosis can successfully be used to treat your pain.

Whatever treatment is chosen to treat RSD, the most important consideration is the rapid diagnosis and institution of treatment to prevent this disease from becoming disabling.

Given that no two people are alike, if you are taking any medications and begin to take nutritional supplements you should be aware that potential drug-nutrient interactions may occur and are encouraged to consult a health care professional before using any natural product. Combining certain prescription drugs and dietary supplements can lead to undesirable effects such as: diminished prescription drug effectiveness, reduced supplement effectiveness and impaired drug and/or supplement absorption.

Probiotic treatment has been shown to improve bone formation, increase bone mass density and prevent bone loss. A study aimed to assess the effect of probiotic treatment on functional recovery in elderly patients with a distal radius fracture.[1] They were randomized to receive skimmed milk containing either a commercial probiotic (Lactobacillus casei Shirota) or placebo daily for a period of 6 months after a fracture. In elderly patients with a fracture of the distal radius, administration of the probiotic could greatly accelerate the healing process with a decrease in the incidence of CRPS I.

Vitamin C administration may be used as a prophylactic measure to prevent the occurrence of reflex sympathetic dystrophy in patients who undergo surgical treatment of a displaced fracture of the distal radius.[2] Vitamin C has been shown to be effective in preventing CRPS I secondary to wrist fracture, but few data are available with respect to foot and ankle cases. A study demonstrated the effectiveness of vitamin C in preventing CRPS I of the foot and ankle.[3] RSD can be treated with vitamin B12 as well.[4]

References

1.      Lei M, Hua LM, Wang DW. The effect of probiotic treatment on elderly patients with distal radius fracture: a prospective double-blind, placebo-controlled randomised clinical trial. Benef Microbes. 2016:1-8.

2.      Cazeneuve JF, Leborgne JM, Kermad K, Hassan Y. [Vitamin C and prevention of reflex sympathetic dystrophy following surgical management of distal radius fractures]. Acta Orthop Belg. 2002;68(5):481-484.

3.      Besse JL, Gadeyne S, Galand-Desme S, Lerat JL, Moyen B. Effect of vitamin C on prevention of complex regional pain syndrome type I in foot and ankle surgery. Foot Ankle Surg. 2009;15(4):179-182.

4.      Beck H. [The shoulder-hand syndrome & its treatment with vitamin B12]. Medizinische. 1958;3(22):922-924.

# 30. SPORTS PAIN

If you have a sports related injury, usually a muscle, tendon, or ligament is involved. Tendons and ligaments can tear apart or tear away from their attachments. The same holds true for muscles. Your bones can also be injured with physical activity. You can have small fractures in one of your bones that occur with repetitive motions such as running. Usually small fractures in bones heal quickly. The most common bone injuries are stress fractures of your small bones, such as those in your feet.

These stress fractures usually take approximately eight weeks to heal. You can develop an abnormal bone growth about the bone in your heel. This abnormal bone growth, which can be painful, is called a spur. Usually a podiatrist or an orthopedic surgeon may have to remove your bone spur if it causes you significant pain. Muscle pain can occur when muscles are stretched beyond their normal elastic limits. When this happens, it is called a strain.

A scar can develop within an injured muscle. An area in this scar can be a source of pain. The scar can be very tender to touch. Occasionally you may need an injection of the scar with a local anesthetic and steroid. The tender areas in your muscles are called trigger points, and these cause a myofascial pain syndrome. Usually ice or heat over the painful muscle can significantly relieve your pain. Massage therapy can also provide you with significant muscle pain relief as well.

You also have cartilage in your joints. Cartilage is a substance that exists between your bones and can be compressed. This compressive ability makes the cartilage act as a shock absorber in some of your joints. Cartilage allows your bones of your joints such as your knee joints to slide over each other. If you do not have the cartilage, one bone will not easily slide over another bone. You would have increased friction applied to your bones in your join if the cartilage is gone which could cause you significant pain. You can also stretch and injure a tendon, which is called a sprain.

An acute sprain is a stretch of a ligament at the time of your injury. If you don't heal within six weeks, you are showing signs of chronic pain. If you still have pain after six months, you have chronic pain. A tendon is composed of a group of fibers that attaches your muscles to your bones. A tendon is composed of tough fibers. A tendon injury can take a long time to heal. Muscle injuries, on the other hand, can heal faster than tendon injuries.

A tendon injury can be potentially serious because if it does not heal properly you can be prone to re-injury. This inflammatory process is called tendonitis.

Some people have bursitis of their shoulders, whereas others may have a bursitis in their hips. A bursa is a sac that is filled with fluid. This fluid-filled sac is placed between either a tendon or a bone or between a ligament and a bone. A bursa allows a tendon to glide over the bone of your shoulder or hip. The fluid is a lubricant. If your bursa becomes inflamed you have bursitis. The covering over your muscle is called a fascia.

The fascia is a tissue that covers your muscles and separates one muscle from another. The fascia is present throughout your body. This fascia enables one muscle to slide smoothly over another muscle. One bone from your upper arm and two bones from your forearm form your elbow joint. You can have irritation of your elbow joint. An injury to your elbow is usually in the tendons of the muscles that attach to the bones about your elbow. In tennis elbow, the pain runs to your outer elbow.

You may also have pain about your inner elbow. This usually occurs when you play golf. Tennis elbow was named because it affected tennis players. However, anyone can develop a tennis elbow. If you have pain on the outside of your elbow, you should stop the activity that caused your pain. You should apply ice over the elbow. Nonsteroidal anti-inflammatory drugs may help you control your pain. If not, you will be referred to an orthopedic surgeon. You should gradually resume your activities.

Inner elbow pain is called golfer's elbow. If you are scrubbing a floor vigorously, you can develop pain in your inner elbow. The pain usually starts several days after you were doing an activity. The treatment for golfer's elbow is the same as that for tennis elbow. You may also develop pain in your elbow joint. Nonsteroidal anti-inflammatory medications will help this pain. Rarely will you need a steroid injection into the joint. You can also develop a bursitis in your elbow.

You can develop a sudden red, swollen area over your elbow. Your range of motion (bending, turning) of your elbow will be normal. Your doctor may want to use a needle and syringe to remove the fluid from your bursa (a process called "aspiration") and send the fluid to a laboratory to test for crystals, bacteria, and so on. If your tests deter-mine that you have gout, you will be treated appropriately. Injection of a steroid into your bursa can provide you with pain relief. If your pain persists, you will be referred to an orthopedic surgeon. Usually ice and nonsteroidal anti-inflammatory drugs will control this pain.

You have many muscles in your arm and around your shoulder. On occasion you can injure your shoulder muscle (rotator cuff muscle) if you fall on your arm and shoulder. You will need to consult with an orthopedic surgeon for treatment. Not every patient with a rotator cuff tear requires surgery. You may only require a steroid injection or a steroid injection followed by physical therapy.

Your knee is made up of your thigh- bone (femur) and your shin-bones (tibia and fibula). There is also a bone in front of your knee called the kneecap (patella). Ligaments hold your bones about your knee together. There is a ligament at either side of your knee. These ligaments provide your knee with stability. Your knee also contains cartilage, which coats your bones. Your cartilage allows your bones to slide over each other with ease. If your cartilage wears out, it can cause you to have arthritis. Between your thigh bone and your shin bone is another cartilage called a meniscus. These cartilages are attached to your shin-bone (tibia).

You also have muscles that control your knee range of motion. These are called the quadriceps and hamstring muscles. When your quadriceps muscles contract, they make your knee straighten. When your hamstring muscles contract, these muscles make your knee and lower leg pull backward at the knee joint. To cushion your knee, you have several bursas in your knee. The ligaments about your knee give your knee stability while the meniscus is a cushion for your knee. Without your meniscus, you would have bone rubbing on bone that would be painful. You can have several areas of pain within your knee including your joint and kneecap. An injury to any one of these anatomic structures can cause you to have knee pain.

If your meniscus degenerates, you will have the loss of the cushion in your knee. This condition is seen in osteoarthritis. If your case is severe you may need a replacement of your joint with an artificial joint.

Hyaluronidase injected into your knee joint may help you with your pain as well as your range of motion. This will consist of several weekly injections. Sometimes these injections can decrease the need for surgery. When doing therapy for your knees, your doctor and physical therapist may emphasize strengthening of the musculature about your joints as opposed to doing extensive knee joint range of motion exercises. If your pain increases during therapy, you need to inform your therapist so that less vigorous therapy can be done.

An X-ray of your knee may show signs of osteoarthritis in the joint where your patella meets your femur. Injection of a local anesthetic about this area can be diagnostic of your disease. Arthroscopy, which involves inserting a scope into your knee, can identify the pathology affecting your knee. If you have pain in your knee, you should apply ice and elevate your knee. You should avoid squatting as well as kneeling. Swimming is preferred to jogging or any impact exercises. You may want to use a Velcro strap around your knee. You should take a nonsteroidal anti-inflammatory medication following your injury.

If you still have pain after two weeks, your doctor may want to aspirate any swelling about your knee. If you still have pain at four weeks, you will probably be referred to an orthopedic surgeon. You need to be aware that a knee injury can predispose you to premature arthritis. Physical therapy does not play an important role in the treatment of a cartilage tear. Sometimes a steroid injection into your knee will prove helpful.

Your hip is a ball and socket joint (figure 3). Hip pain is common problem as well, and its source of pain can be confusing because there are many causes. It is important to make an accurate diagnosis of the cause of your symptoms so that appropriate treatment can be directed at the underlying hip problem. Arthritis is among the most frequent causes of hip pain.

Trochanteric bursitis is an extremely common problem that causes inflammation of the bursa over the outside of your hip joint. A steroid injection into your knee can provide you with pain relief. Tendonitis can occur in any of the tendons that surround your hip joint. A nonsteroidal anti-inflammatory medication may provide you with pain relief or you may need a steroid injection.

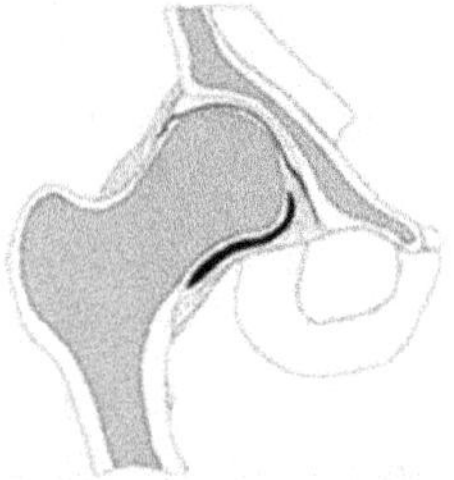

Figure 1. The hip joint is a ball and socket joint.

Osteonecrosis is a condition that occurs when blood flow to an area of your hip- bone is restricted. If an inadequate amount of blood flow reaches your bone, the cells will die and your bone may collapse. One of the most common places for osteonecrosis to occur is in your hip joint. Hip fractures are most common in elderly patients. These fractures usually require surgery. A disc herniation in your lower back may refer pain to your hip as well.

An ankle sprain is a partial tear of the ligaments of your ankle joint. In a Grade I sprain your ligament is intact. In a Grade II, your ligament is partially torn and in a Grade III tear, your ligament is completely torn. Your ligaments can be pulled away from the location where they attach to your bones.

A sprain can be classified as acute, recurrent, or chronic. In an acute injury, your range of motion about your ankle will be limited. With chronic pain, your range of motion will be greater. Chronic instability of your ankle could lead to a decreased range of motion about your ankle as well as pain with motion. As a result, you may develop arthritis of your ankle.

If your pain persists for a prolonged period, your doctor may have you do physical therapy and may possibly prescribe an orthotic for you (to be placed in your shoe). Remember that you should see your doctor if your acute injury does not resolve in four to seven days. Your primary care doctor may even refer you to an orthopedic surgeon. Steroid injections may provide you with relief if other modalities fail. You may need x-rays of your ankle to exclude a tear of your ligament from your bone. Upon examination of the x-ray, your doctor may notice small flecks of bone.

If your pain persists beyond your normal healing time, a magnetic resonance imaging (MRI) scan may be necessary. The overall goal of treatment is to allow your injury to heal. As previously stated, immediately after the injury you should apply ice and rest the ankle. You should also limit weight bearing.

You can immobilize your ankle with an Ace wrap. You may need to temporarily use a crutch. Usually after a week or two you can begin to do some stretching exercises. You may need to wear a Velcro ankle brace or high-top tennis shoes at this time. You should not engage in stop-and-go sports such as basketball, running, or impact aerobics. You must realize that injury healing is measured in months rather than weeks.

You have a strong ligament that attaches the muscle of your calf to your heel. This tendon is called your Achilles tendon. Your foot has tendons and muscles that help pull your toes downward or pull your toes upward toward. The tendon attaches your calf muscle to your ankle. An x-ray will not help with the diagnosis of an Achilles tendonitis.

An MRI scan will help with the diagnosis. Following and injury ibuprofen may help your pain. You may need an ankle brace. If your pain persists more than six weeks, you may need high-top tennis shoes. You should increase your activities gradually if your pain persists.

If pain persists more than two weeks, see an orthopedic surgeon. An injection with a steroid may provide with some relief. However, realize that physical therapy plays an important role in this type of injury. If pain persists, you may need surgery.

You also have a bursa about your Achilles tendon as well. This bursa can become inflamed. If this occurs, you will have pain in the back of your heel. X-rays are not helpful in the diagnosis of a bursitis in this area. Usually the diagnosis is made if you have pain immediately above your heel. An injection of local anesthetic in this area can confirm the diagnosis. Your doctor may apply a steroid. Injection may be repeated. You should have physical therapy. Occasionally your doctor may want to immobilize your ankle.

Exercise may cause you to have shoulder pain. You may also sustain a rotator cuff tendon tear if you fall on an outstretched arm or if you are frequently using your arm for vigorous activity. This tendon attaches a muscle to the bone in your upper arm called the humerus. A tear in this tendon can cause weakness and pain in your shoulder. You may sustain this injury if you fall or do violent pulls on a starter cable.

Excessive pushing and pulling can cause tears as well. These tears usually respond to stretch exercises as well as nonsteroidal anti-inflammatory medications. On occasion, you may need an injection with a steroid. If you do not respond to conservative care within four weeks, see an orthopedic surgeon. If you have a moderate to large rotator cuff tendon tear, you are a probable candidate for surgery. You will need to be evaluated by an ortho-pedic surgeon.

Injections with steroids are commonly done for the following musculo-skeletal disorders. Injection of the sub acromial space for treatment of rotator cuff tendinitis and shoulder impingement syndrome is a com-mon and useful injection. This technique also can be used diagnostically to differentiate between shoulder joint and cervical spine pain.

The long head of your biceps tendon often is irritated by overuse. Anesthetic injection of the peritendinous space can help confirm the diagno-sis of biceps tendinitis.

The pes anserine bursa is located along the medial aspect of the knee joint about 2 cm below the medial joint line. It is a common site of irritation that results in painful tendinitis or bursitis.

The prepatellar bursa often becomes irritated. It is superficial to the patella and easily palpable when swollen. Aspiration of a swollen bursa can provide symptomatic relief and is required for fluid analysis. Intra-articular aspiration or injection of the knee is indicated to obtain fluid for analysis, treat painful osteoarthritis, or relieve a tense effusion.

De Quervain's tenosynovitis is a painful condition of the thumb and wrist that can be treated with a corticosteroid injection. Injection is indicated for treatment of the carpal tunnel syndrome when less invasive treatments are unsuccessful.

A dorsal ganglion of the wrist that has become painful or irritated may be aspirated and injected. Lateral epicondylitis may be treated by injection when less invasive treatments have failed. Injection has been shown to provide short-term relief. Treatment of olecranon bursitis with aspiration and injection closely parallels treatment of prepatellar bursitis.

Bursitis of the greater trochanter of the femur is painful and often responds well to corticosteroid injection. An anesthetic injection also is useful to differentiate between local pain and referred pain. Plantar fasciitis of the foot may be treated with an injection as well. Trigger point injections may be used to treat many painful soft-tissue conditions.

Given that no two people are alike, if you are taking any medications and begin to take nutritional supplements you should be aware that potential drug-nutrient interactions may occur and are encouraged to consult a health care professional before using any natural product. Combining certain prescription drugs and dietary supplements can lead to undesirable effects such as: diminished prescription drug effectiveness, reduced supplement effectiveness and impaired drug and/or supplement absorption.

It is well recognized that vitamin D is necessary for optimal bone health. Evidence is finding that vitamin D deficiency can have a profound effect on immunity, inflammation and muscle function. Dietary assessment studies have found that athletes worldwide do not meet the dietary intake recommendations for vitamin D, the most probable reason for poor status is inadequate synthesis due to lack of sun exposure.

Studies in athletic populations suggest that maintaining adequate vitamin D status may reduce stress fractures, total body inflammation, common infectious illnesses, and impaired muscle function, and may also aid in recovery from injury.[1]

Vitamin D is well known for its role in calcium regulation and bone health, but emerging literature tells of vitamin D's central role in other vital body processes, such as: signaling gene response, protein synthesis, hormone synthesis, immune response, plus, cell turnover and regeneration. The discovery of the vitamin D receptor within the muscle suggested a significant role for vitamin D in muscle tissue function.[2]

Adequate nutrition plays an important role in the development and maintenance of bone structures resistant to usual mechanical stresses. In addition to calcium in the presence of an adequate supply of vitamin D, dietary proteins represent key nutrients for bone health and thereby function in the prevention of osteoporosis. Several studies point to a positive effect of high protein intake on bone mineral density or content. This fact is associated with a significant reduction in hip fracture incidence in postmenopausal women.[3]

Physical activities that improve muscular strength, endurance, and balance may reduce fracture risk by reducing the risk of falling. The combined effect of physical activity and calcium supplementation on bone mineral needs further investigation.[4] Protein and calcium intake should be considered in the prevention or treatment of the chronic diseases osteoporosis and sarcopenia.[5] protein intake in the elderly in Europe that may furthermore result in increased bone loss and risk of osteoporotic fracture.[6]

References

1.        Larson-Meyer E. Vitamin D supplementation in athletes. Nestle Nutr Inst Workshop Ser. 2013;75:109-121.

2.        Ogan D, Pritchett K. Vitamin D and the athlete: risks, recommendations, and benefits. Nutrients. 2013;5(6):1856-1868.

3.        Bonjour JP. Protein intake and bone health. Int J Vitam Nutr Res. 2011;81(2-3):134-142.

4.        Lewis RD, Modlesky CM. Nutrition, physical activity, and bone health in women. Int J Sport Nutr. 1998;8(3):250-284.

5.        Genaro Pde S, Martini LA. Effect of protein intake on bone and muscle mass in the elderly. Nutr Rev. 2010;68(10):616-623.

6.        Ginty F. Dietary protein and bone health. Proc Nutr Soc. 2003;62(4):867-876.

# 31. HIV

The acquired immune deficiency syndrome (AIDS) is caused by the human immunodeficiency virus (HIV). The virus can replicate itself within a host cell or do nothing once it infects the host cell. When a virus replicates itself in a host cell, thousands or even millions of copies of itself can be released from the cell and then go on to infect other cells. HIV, for example, can enter your body from unsafe sex practices or contaminated blood, enter your cells, and make millions, billions, and even trillions of copies of itself that go on to infect other cells in your body.

A virus, therefore, is a highly effective means of causing you to develop and have an infection. If the virus gets into your body, it can cause a disease unless your antibodies attack it. A virus, on the other hand, can reproduce only by invading one of your cells.

A virus is spread randomly through the wind, in water, food, by blood, or by body secretions. With respect to HIV, blood and body secretions are important mechanisms by which this virus spreads from one person's body into our body. HIV, which is the causative virus of AIDS, is a very complex virus.

When new viruses are replicated, the virus that destroys the outer wall of your cell releases an enzyme. The enzyme destroys the outer wall of your cell. When this wall is destroyed, the new viruses that have been made within your cell are now released into your body.

These viruses will go to infect other cells of different tissues within your body. As this process progresses, you will develop fever, chills, joint pain, nerve and muscle pain, and so forth.

Be aware that when the new virus is made from the original virus, your cell that was infected by the virus will then be destroyed. When a new virus infects your cell, it does not cause immediate cellular destruction. This example is the reason why HIV can be present in the body for some time before causing symptoms. You can become infected with the HIV virus by exposure to infected blood products, sexual contact with infected people, or from a mother to her baby.

Infection from this virus appears within two to six weeks following infection. Early symptoms of infection with HIV are much like flu symptoms and include muscle pain, joint pain, headaches, as well as a sore throat and fever. Antibodies to the HIV virus develop in your body within three to six months of your infection. Later symptoms, which take up to 10 years to develop, as those of AIDS, result from the destructive effects of HIV on your immune system and are characterized by unusual types of pneumonia, cancer, central nervous system infections, and other problems.

Changes in your immune system will eventually occur after you have been infected. After the HIV virus enters your cells, each virus can set up a chronic infection in which new virus particles are constantly being produced. You may develop some antibodies to the virus. When the level of your body's antibodies decreases, you can develop AIDS.

Progression to AIDS, which is a syndrome following infection with the virus, can begin with a low red blood cell count. Other factors can be necessary for you to contract the HIV infection and for the development of progression to AIDS.

There are four high-risk groups for acquiring AIDS; homosexual and bisexual men, hemophiliacs and transfusion recipients, intravenous drug abusers and children born to infected mothers. Homosexual and bisexual men account for approximately 37-40 percent of the reported cases of AIDS in the United States. However, this number is increasing. The majority of women with AIDS in the United States are in childbearing years.

The number of individuals with AIDS does not take into account the high number of HIV-infected asymptomatic women. Remember that an HIV infection takes time to develop AIDS. The risks for a woman to expose herself to the HIV virus are through unsafe sex practices, intravenous drug use, and transfusions. A significant number of HIV-infected women have given birth to HIV-infected babies.

There is speculation that pregnancy can accelerate the disease pro-gres-sion of HIV. If you are pregnant and have HIV, you may develop symptoms two to three years after the delivery of your baby. This rate of AIDS development is faster than for homosexual men or intravenous drug users; approximately 40 percent of asymptomatic carriers of the virus in these categories will develop AIDS.

The AIDS virus will decrease your lymphocytes, which are cells that normally exist in your bloodstream. Lymphocytes are important mediators of your immune system. These cells help fight the development of various diseases. The average time of onset of your viral infection to development of AIDS varies months to years with a mean time of approximately 10 years.

Health-care providers cannot test an individual for HIV without permission. To test for an HIV infection, your doctor must obtain an informed consent from you. Informed consent is a legal requirement and means that your doctor must inform you that you will be tested for HIV.

You must sign an agreement that gives your doctor the right to do this test. Without your informed consent, your doctor is violating your patient rights.

The name for the initial viral test performed is ELISA (enzyme-linked immune absorbent assay). If you have a positive screening test using ELISA, the infection with the HIV complex is confirmed with a repeat ELISA test as well as another test called a Western blot test. A doctor will usually not report a positive ELISA test to you until your Western blot test has been confirmed to be positive.

The HIV virus induces AIDS by causing the death of the CD4+T cells in your body. These cells are important for the normal function of your immune system. The AIDS virus also interferes with their normal function. When this happens, your ability to fight other infections is diminished. HIV virus is called a slow virus. This means that the course of infection with the HIV virus has a long interval between the initial infection and the onset of the AIDS symptoms.

HIV/AIDS can cause: fever and night sweats, loss of appetite, nausea and vomiting, chest pain related to pneumonia, chronic sinus infection with headache, tumor on your spinal cord, meningitis with neck pain and headaches, painful lesions in your mouth, hepatitis with abdominal pain and/or, burning or piercing pain in your arms or legs

Once infected, you can progress to AIDS in an average of 10 years as previously mentioned. Combinations of three or more anti-HIV drugs called highly active antiretroviral therapy can delay the progression of the HIV disease for prolonged periods. This disease frequently causes a painful neuropathy in many areas of your body. A neuropathy is a lesion in your nerves in your body that are outside of your spinal cord and brain.

AIDS can cause you to have a painful neuropathy. Neuropathy associ-ated with AIDS can be intermittent or constant. The pain can vary in severity from mild to severe. The pain can be burning, shooting, aching, or stabbing. It is believed that the HIV virus causes nerve damage, which causes your painful neuropathy. You can develop headaches from HIV virus meningitis. Also you can have abdominal pain related to gastrointestinal disease and chest pain related to pneumonia.

You may develop headaches as well as fever and have significant changes in your mental status as your infection progresses. To make this diagnosis, your doctor will do a spinal tap by placing a needle into your spinal fluid. The laboratory will identify any abnormal cells in your spinal fluid. Your doctor will measure your spinal fluid pressure by placing a needle into your spinal fluid to see whether you are having excessive pressure on your brain. You may need repeated spinal fluid taps followed by removal of some of your spinal fluid to decrease any pressure that could be affecting your brain.

One of the leading causes of death in individuals with AIDS is the pneumocystis carini pneumonia. This is the most common infection in AIDS patients and is the leading cause of death in this patient population. Not only does this disease affect your lungs, it can affect other parts of your body as well. If you have AIDS, you can also develop tumors associated with AIDS. These tumors include Kaposi's sarcoma as well as Hodgkin's and non-Hodgkins lymphoma.

There is now hope for individuals infected with HIV. It is estimated that if 1 million people in the United States now have HIV or AIDS, approximately 500,000 of them are either untreated or undiagnosed. Drugs for the treatment of AIDS are constantly being developed. Essentially, AIDS has gone from being an immediate sentence of death to a chronic manageable disease. Currently Russia has the fastest growing epidemic of AIDS, thought to be because of intravenous drug use. Epidemics are now beginning in China.

The rate of AIDS cases and deaths did slowdown, which was attributed to successful antiretroviral therapy. The problem with some of the drug therapy is that some individuals either develop a resistance to the drugs or they experience side effects from the drugs and stop taking them. Some of the vaccines currently being studied provide protection for some individuals but not all. Two anti-HIV drugs have been shown to cause eath in some pregnant women. These drugs are stavudine and didanosine. Between 1991 and 1995, there was a 63 percent increase in women diagnosed with AIDS.

Your pain can be treated with narcotic drugs as well as antidepressants and anticonvulsant medications such as Neurontin. Intravenous lidocaine may decrease your pain. Mexilitine, a heart rhythm medication, may also help to control your pain. Exercise therapy is sometimes beneficial for the management of your pain. It is believed that exercise can increase your body's endorphins, which in turn helps to manage your pain.

Endorphins are natural chemical substances that your body produces HIV-related pain becomes increasingly severe as the disease progresses. Drugs used to treat the HIV infection can cause neuropathic pain. It is estimated that 30 percent of the neuropathic pain syndromes suffered by individuals who have the HIV disease are caused by drugs to attack the HIV virus. Neuropathic pain in the HIV-infected patient in most instances can be adequately controlled.

Given that no two people are alike, if you are taking any medications and begin to take nutritional supplements you should be aware that potential drug-nutrient interactions may occur and are encouraged to consult a health care professional before using any natural product. Combining certain prescription drugs and dietary supplements can lead to undesirable effects such as: diminished prescription drug effectiveness, reduced supplement effectiveness and impaired drug and/or supplement absorption.

Food insecurity is defined as a limited or uncertain ability to acquire acceptable foods in socially acceptable ways, or limited or uncertain availability of nutritionally adequate and safe foods. Improvement in life expectancy with the use of combination antiretroviral therapy has come with the recognition of the complications associated with chronic human immunodeficiency virus infection. Vitamin D has been of particular interest because of its effect on bone health and immune functions. Vitamin D deficiency was common among the patients included in this study.[1]

A study was done to determine the effects of nutritional status at the start of highly active anti-retroviral therapy on treatment outcomes. Malnutrition predisposes HIV patients to early death.[2]

The response to the HIV infection is situated within complex interactions between host nutritional health and immunologic function, which contribute to the varied phenotypes of immune activation among HIV-infected patients across a spectrum from malnutrition to obesity.[3]

HIV patients who experienced severe food insecurity negatively influenced their mental health and general wellbeing. The inclusion of resources for food assistance in HIV treatment programs may help ameliorate mental health challenges.[4]

References

1.      Mirza A, Wells S, Gayton T, et al. Vitamin D Deficiency in HIV-Infected Children. South Med J. 2016;109(11):683-687.

2.      Hussen S, Belachew T, Hussien N. Nutritional status and its effect on treatment outcome among HIV infected clients receiving HAART in Ethiopia: a cohort study. AIDS Res Ther. 2016;13:32.

3.      Koethe JR, Heimburger DC, PrayGod G, Filteau S. From Wasting to Obesity: The Contribution of Nutritional Status to Immune Activation in HIV Infection. J Infect Dis. 2016;214 Suppl 2:S75-82.

4.      Hatsu I, Hade E, Campa A. Food Security Status is Related to Mental Health Quality of Life Among Persons Living with HIV. AIDS Behav. 2016.

Cancer pain is usually not evident until the cancer growth has become far advanced. Most non-solid tumors cause minimal pain while solid tumors like prostate cancer can cause significant pain. If you have myeloma, you will have a malignant formation of your plasma cells.

Plasma cells are antibody-producing cells found in bone forming tissue as well as in your lungs and your abdomen. This increase in your plasma cells can affect your organs and cause you to have painful symptoms. Usually bone pain is the most common pain noted involving multiple myeloma.

Multiple myeloma can be an extremely painful entity affecting your bones and is usually treated by a medical specialist who treats cancer called an oncologist.

Lung cancer is common in the United States. Lung Cancer is a disease that begins in the tissue of the lungs. Oxygen is taken up by your body and carbon dioxide is removed. The vast majority of lung cancer cases fall into one of two different categories: Non-Small Cell Lung Cancer is the most common type of lung cancer, making up nearly 80% of all cases.

This type of lung cancer grows and spreads more slowly than small cell lung cancer. Small Cell Lung Cancer makes up nearly 20% of all lung cancer cases.

It is associated with cancer cells smaller than most other cancer cells. These cells may be small, but they can rapidly reproduce to form large tumors. Their size and quick rate of reproduction allows them to spread to the lymph nodes and to other organs of the body. Cigarette smoking causes this type of cancer.

Symptoms of lung cancer include the following: coughing, shortness of breath, wheezing, pain in your chest, shoulder, upper back, or arm, coughing up blood, frequent pneumonia, generalized pain and hoarse-ness. Lung cancer can spread to your brain liver or bone.

As a result, you may experience headaches, seizures, abdominal pain or bone pain. Non-small cell lung cancer can be treated with surgery while small cell cancer is treated with chemotherapy. Sometimes, a small segment of the lung can be removed while in other cases, the whole lobe must be removed.

Colon cancer is another common cancer that you need to be aware of. The colon is the part of your body where the waste material is stored. The rectum is the end of the colon adjacent to the anus. Together, they form a long, muscular tube called the large intestine (also known as the large bowel). Tumors of the colon and rectum are growths arising from the inner wall of the large intestine. Benign tumors of the large intestine are called polyps. Malignant tumors of the large intestine are called cancers. Cancer of the colon and rectum (also referred to as colorectal cancer) can invade and damage adjacent tissues and organs. Cancer cells can also break away and spread to other parts of the body (such as your liver and lung.

Factors that increase a person's risk of colorectal cancer include high fat intake, a family history of colorectal cancer and polyps, the presence of polyps in the large intestine, and chronic ulcerative colitis.

Symptoms of colon cancer are usually nonspecific. They include: fatigue, weakness, and shortness of breath, change in bowel habits, bloody stools, diarrhea and/ or constipation, blood in your stool, weight loss, abdominal pain or cramps. If colon cancer is suspected a barium enema X ray or a colonoscopy will be done.

Surgery is the most common treatment for cancer of the rectum and colon. If the cancer has spread you may also require chemotherapy. If your cancer is limited to your rectum, you may be treated with radiation therapy.

Some cancers can be gender specific. For example, if you are a female, you can develop cancer of your breasts, cervix, uterus, or ovary. If you are male, you can develop cancer of your testicles, prostate gland or breast. Cancer-related pain can be excruciating in some cases.

Various treatment methods and therapies are available to help relieve your pain if it is caused by a cancer. Breast cancer is the most common malignancy in women in the United States. Approximately 182,000 women develop breast cancer and more than 46,000 die with it. It occurs in one in eight women. Approximate-ly two thirds of cases occur after menopause. Fifteen percent of cases occur before the age of 40. Screening for female cancers is very important.

The actual cause of breast cancer is not known. There are different types of breast cancer. Some breast cancers can affect the ducts of the breasts, whereas other types affect the lobules of the breasts.

Cancer of the ducts usually occurs on one side of the body, whereas lobular cancer is bilateral. You must be taught how to do self-examination of your breasts. The majority of women detect their own breast cancer. You should have a breast examination by your doctor at the time of your regular physical examination if you are over age 40. Mammography is recommended every 1 to 2 years if you are older than 40 years of age.

If you have a history of breast cancer, you should have a mammogram yearly. If you are over 40 and have a family history of breast cancer, you should also have a mammogram every year. The survival rate is lower if your cancer is detected by a mammogram as opposed to palpation. Breast cancer is usually painless and presents with a palpable mass in a postmenopausal woman. If it had associated pain, the diagnosis would be earlier diagnosed. You should perform routine self-examinations as your cancer can be diagnosed early as opposed to waiting for your doctor or mammogram to make the diagnosis.

An accurate diagnosis of breast cancer requires a needle aspiration, a percutaneous needle biopsy, or an incisional (surgical) biopsy. A biopsy should be done on every suspicious breast mass. You must have a chest x-ray to see if your breast cancer may have spread to your lungs, ribs, or spine. A bone scan may also be required to see if your breast cancer has spread to your bones. If you have breast cancer, your doctor will want to get a CAT scan of your abdomen to see if the cancer has affected your liver as well.

Your doctor will also obtain a liver function test from you because your cancer can spread to your liver. Risks for breast cancer include increasing age, a family history of breast cancer, previous cancer in one breast, early menstruation (meaning before age 12), late menopause (meaning after age 52), a history of having no children, obesity, a high fat diet, alcohol use, and a family history of cancer of the ovary, uterus, or colon.

A pathologist will stage your cancer. Staging determines the severity of your cancer. A 0 stage cancer is confined to an area of your organ. A stage greater than III usually means that the cancer has spread beyond your organ. Your survival rate depends on the stage of the cancer. The stages are based on the severity of the cancer.

The higher the stage correlates with a lower survival rate. If you have cancer in your breast that has not spread to your bones or other organs, your 5-year survival rate is greater than 95 percent. However, if your cancer has spread to other areas of your body, your 5-year survival rate is only 10 percent. If your cancer is only in your tissue, you may only need removal of that part of the tissue from your breast.

Cancer treatment is complex and new methods are frequently being developed to treat advanced metastatic cancer. However, you are encouraged to do your own breast exams. This may help you to discover the cancer much earlier than if you wait to have an exam at your yearly physical examination or during a mammogram.

If your breast cancer has spread to other areas of your body, you will most likely require a mastectomy (removal of your breast, radiation therapy, chemotherapy, as well as hormone therapy).

Your oncologist will discuss with you the best options for your treatment. Breast cancer can also occur in males. Males can have an enlargement of their breast tissue.

Estrogens stimulate breast development. Androgens such as testosterone inhibit breast development. Male breast cancer is usually on one side and presents as a firm mass that appears to be fixed to the male's underlying muscle. There may even be a nipple discharge. There may also be retraction of the skin around the male breast.

With respect to female cancer, cervical cancer accounts for approximately 2 to 3 percent of all cancers involving women in the United States. More than 15,000 cases of cervical cancer are diagnosed each year, and approximately 5,000 women die from this disease. Risk factors for developing carcinoma of the cervix include suppression of the immune system, a history of genital herpes or genital warts, multiple sexual partners, partners with penile warts or cancer, low economic status, intercourse before age 17, and cigarette smoking. Usually cancer of the cervix is painless. A Pap smear detects many cases of cervical cancer.

If you have abnormal vaginal bleeding, vaginal discharge, or bleeding after intercourse, you may have advanced cervical cancer. Cancer from your cervix can spread and can cause you to experience lower back pain, leg pain, weight loss, or swelling in your legs. If you have an abnormal Pap smear, you will have a biopsy of your cervix. If the biopsy is unable to determine whether a suspicious-looking tissue is cancerous, you will have a greater portion of your cervix removed, which is called a cervical conization.

Your doctor will obtain liver function tests from you, a creatinine level, and a squamous cell carcinoma antigen level. A chest x-ray will be obtained to see whether the cancer has spread to your ribs or lungs. An MRI of your pelvis and abdomen will be obtained to see whether the cancer has spread to other organs. Your gynecologist may place a scope in your bladder and one in your sigmoid colon to see whether the cancer has advanced to your gastrointestinal tract or urinary tract.

As with most cancers, a pathologist will assign a numeric stage to your cancer. A high number means that your cancer has spread beyond the organ where it began. If your cancer is only confined to your cervix, you have a 5-year survival rate of 100 percent. If your cancer has spread throughout your pelvis and involved your bladder or rectum, your 5-year survival rate is 20 percent.

If your cancer is in an advanced stage and has spread outside of the cervix to other areas of your body, your oncologist will probably prescribe radiation therapy and possibly chemotherapy. If your cancer has spread to your upper vagina, your gynecological oncologist may elect to do abdominal hysterectomy as well as removal of your lymph nodes. On the other hand, this doctor may elect to do radiation therapy.

Many times the treatment chosen by your doctor depends on your overall health status. After your treatment, your gynecological oncologist will perform a comprehensive pelvic examination as well as a Pap smear every three months for the first two years following your initial treatment. After that, the examination and Pap smear should be every six months from years three to five. If you develop a recurrent cancer of your cervix, you will then probably experience vaginal bleeding or discharge. You can develop pain in your back and legs as well. Again you may experience weight loss. If this happens, you may be treated with radiation therapy or with an extensive removal of the organs in your pelvis.

Approximately 34,000 cases of cancer of the uterus occur each year in the United States. The incidence of this uterine tumor decreases yearly. The death rate has decreased each year since 1950. Usually this cancer will occur if you are a postmenopausal woman. Women who undergo menopause after age 52 are more prone to develop uterine cancer. Obesity contributes to an increase in this type of cancer.

If you are taking estrogen replacement and are over age 52, you have an increased risk of developing uterine cancer. As with the other cancers mentioned in this chapter, there are stages. Stage 0, which is the cancer in your uterus, has a 100 percent success rate. If your cancer involves your bladder or your rectum, your survival rate decreases to 20 percent.

If you have stage 0 uterine cancer, a simple procedure that removes the area of the cancer can be done. If you have the fourth stage, which involves your bladder, pelvis, or rectum, you will have radiation therapy. If you have stage 2A, you will have a radical hysterectomy with removal of your lymph nodes followed by radiation therapy. The clinical presentation of this cancer is abnormal uterine bleeding. If you are in menopause and begin bleeding, your gynecologist or primary care doctor should evaluate you immediately.

If your cancer becomes advanced, you can have pelvic pain as well as back and leg pain. You will also have a weight loss. Almost 5 percent of women with uterine cancer have no symptoms. You should have a careful and comprehensive pelvic and abdominal evaluation. If you have abnormal bleeding, you should have a biopsy taken from your uterus or a D&C. Most of the uterine cancers detected by your doctor are at usually at an early stage. This means that your prognosis for a five-year survival is good.

Standard therapy for uterine cancer is an abdominal hysterectomy with removal of both your ovaries. As with other cancers mentioned in this chapter, you should have a pelvic exam and Pap smear every three months for the first two years after treatment. Other tests should be done only if you have a recurrence of symptoms.

If you do have recurrence of the cancer, a major surgical procedure will need to be done. Ovarian cancer develops in 1 in every 70 women. Approximately 1 percent of women die from this cancer. Approximately 24,000 cases of ovarian cancer are diagnosed in the United States each year. More than 13,000 women will die with ovarian cancer each year.

The incidence of cancer of the ovary is increased in women who have never been pregnant and is more prevalent in women who have had late onset of menopause or have been on a high-fat diet. If you are female and have a history of colon cancer or breast cancer, you are at a higher risk for developing ovarian cancer. If you are using oral contraceptives, have had more than one baby, and are breast-feeding, you will have a decreased risk of developing cancer of the ovaries.

If someone in your family has a history of ovarian cancer, you are at an increased risk. If your cancer is confined to your ovary, you have a stage 1A cancer. You have a five-year survival rate of approximately 90 percent. If you have a stage IV ovarian tumor, the cancer has spread to your liver or lung or so forth. Your five-year survival rate is 5 percent. Unfortunately, most women who have cancer of their ovaries will have an advanced disease at the time of their diagnosis.

The reason for this is that the symptoms of ovarian cancer are vague. You may have vague pelvic or abdominal pain. You may only have altered bowel habits. As your cancer develops, you can have obstruction of your intestines and can have swelling and fluid in your abdomen. Sometimes the tumor can be noted on a routine physical pelvic examination.

You can have abnormal uterine bleeding. If you are a postmenopausal female and if your doctor can palpate your ovary on a routine pelvic exam, this suggests that you may have an ovarian tumor.

Usually, normal ovaries cannot be palpated. If you have an enlarged ovary, an ultrasound of your pelvis may be helpful in diagnosing cancer of your ovary. Your pelvis, abdomen, and chest will be carefully examined as well. Liver-function tests will be done as well as a CAT scan of your abdomen. Occasionally a further gastrointestinal workup is indicated.

If you have ovarian cancer, you will have your ovaries removed as well as your uterus. You will also have surgical sampling of your lymph glands to see whether your cancer has spread to your lymph glands. Chemotherapy may be prescribed to your after surgery. Your prognosis is good if you are relatively young and if you have an early stage of the cancer and if you have a rapid rate of your ovarian tumor response to the therapy mentioned.

As we have seen with all of these tumors, the higher the number of the stage, the worse the tumor (Stage III is worse than II). If you have an extremely malignant tumor, your prognosis of survival over five years may be poor. This is the reason that you must get your gynecological examination on a regular basis. The reason for this is that if your tumor is diagnosed early, you have an excellent survival prognosis.

Males suffer from gender specific tumors as well. The testes secrete testosterone and estradiol, which are two hormones. Testicular cancer represents approximately 2 percent of all cancers in men. It is the second most common cancer in men between the ages of 20 and 34 years of age.

These tumors usually manifest as an enlargement of the testicle. You may have pain and tenderness in your testicle. A male with a testicular tumor can have breast enlargement. Approximately 10 percent of these tumors will have distant spread of the cancer at the time of the diagnosis.

These tumors are staged through measurement of certain chemical markers in the bloodstream as well as imaging studies or surgery. Some of these cancers are quite sensitive to radiation therapy.

Other tumors that are confined to the testes are cured through removal of the testicle followed by radiation therapy. If your tumor has spread throughout your body, the disease is treated with both radiation therapy and chemotherapy. If your cancer is localized to your testicle, your 5-year survival rate approximates 100 percent. If your cancer has spread throughout your body, your survival rate drops to 20 percent.

Most men over 55 years of age may have an enlargement of their prostate gland. Almost two thirds of these men will have symptoms of prostatism. They will have decreased force of their urine stream and retention of their urine in their bladder after they urinate. They wake up frequently at night to urinate.

Over time, they may not be able to hold their urine. Prostatism is a benign entity. However, prostatism can be a symptom of cancer. Cancer symptoms may be without significant symptoms initially but as the cancer advances can become severe.

Prostate cancer is the second most common tumor in men. Lung cancer is the most common. Approximately 200,000 new cases are diagnosed each year in the United States. Prostate cancer is more common among African Americans and men who have a family history of prostate cancer.

The problem with prostate cancer is that it is usually painless and has no other symptoms that are seen with prostatism. Prostate cancer can be detected by routine digital examination or elevation of your prostate specific antigen (PSA). Sometimes if you have surgery to remove an enlarged prostate gland, cancer tissue can be found in your prostate gland.

When the cancer travels from your prostate gland and goes to your bone, you can have severe back pain or other bone pain. In many instances, an MRI will be done to see whether your tumor has spread to other organs. Other chemical body markers can be measured as well if cancer is suspected to be present in another organ.

A bone scan may be necessary to detect a cancer that has gone to your bones. If you have prostate cancer, your surgeon may do a prostatectomy (removal of your prostate gland), radiation therapy, hormone therapy, or chemotherapy.

If your tumor is confined to your prostate, a prostatectomy, radiation therapy and/or hormone therapy may be necessary. If your prostate cancer has spread beyond your prostate, radiation therapy is usually the treatment of choice. If your prostate cancer has disseminated throughout your body, you will be treated with hormone therapy.

Your prostate cancer is usually testosterone sensitive. Your doctor will prescribe hormone therapy that will lower your testosterone in your bloodstream. This can be done through castration.

Your doctor can give you large doses of estrogen, which will eventual-ly lower your testosterone blood level. Chemotherapy is usually not effective for the management of prostate cancer. Following treatment, your PSA will be monitored regularly to determine the effects of your therapy. If your PSA continues to rise, this indicates probable residual cancer.

Prostate cancer can be detected early; if it is detected early, your prognosis for survival is excellent. This means that you need to follow up with your primary care doctor regularly and have a regular rectal examination so that your doctor can feel your prostate to see if it is enlarged or if it has possible cancer masses in it. You will also need to have your PSA done on a regular basis.

There is no reason why cancer pain cannot be controlled. There are multiple modalities now available to adequately control cancer pain.

If you have been diagnosed with cancer, you face a wide range of psychological and physical problems throughout your cancer. You may have a fear of a painful death or disfigurement. One of the most feared conse-quences of cancer is pain. To treat your pain appropriately, a multidisciplinary approach may be necessary, including your oncologist, your psychologist or psychiatrist, and your pain-management doctor.

Almost 90 percent of psychiatric disorders noted in cancer patients are a reaction to the disease itself or treatments used to cure the cancer. An extremely painful disease is the most feared effect associated with cancer.

Approximately 15 percent of cancer patients whose cancer has not spread develop significant pain. If the disease is advanced, 60 to 90 percent of patients report significant pain. Unfortunately, 25 percent of all cancer patients die while still experiencing considerable pain.

As your tumor grows it can compress nerves in areas of your body, which can cause you pain. Your cancer pain can cause you sharp, aching, and throbbing pain as well.

Pain from your organs is more diffuse as well as gnawing and cramping. Most of your pain can respond to narcotic drugs. If your pain is in your central nervous system or if it affects some of your nerves outside of your brain and spinal cord, you can have what is called neuropathic pain.

Neuropathic pain causes you to experience symptoms that are sharp and electrical shock like. This type of pain can be controlled by antiseizure medications such as Neurontin or Lyrica. You can have pain that is severe and excessive for the extent of tissue damage that has occurred. This type of pain is called idiopathic and usually has a psychological pathology associated with it.

Anticonvulsant medications can relieve severe lancinating pain when your tumor affects one of your nerves. In case you are wondering why a seizure medication would be prescribed, it's because these medications are also pain medications. In the United States, about 5 percent of all anticonvulsant medications are prescribed for pain management.

Nerve injury caused by cancer, chemotherapy, or radiation therapy is controlled with anticonvulsant medications. Nonsteroidal anti-inflammatory medications may relieve bone pain related to your cancer.

Narcotics can relieve your cancer pain. Morphine is the standard of comparison for the rest of the narcotic analgesics. A sustained-release preparation is available called MS Contin releases the drug over 8 to 12 hours. Oxycontin also provides a release of oxycodone over 8-12 hours. There is also a drug that you can take once a day that will give a sustained release over 24 hours called Kadian.

Dilaudid is stronger than morphine, but it has a shorter duration of action than morphine. Methadone is another drug that can be prescribed for cancer pain. It is very effective when given in a pill form. Another drug more potent than morphine is Levo-Dromoran. It is stronger than morphine and can last up to 16 hours per dose. Opana, a long acting oxymorphone is also available.

Fentanyl is a potent drug that is more potent than the drugs mentioned. A transdermal fentanyl patch gives you a continuous dose of drug. There is also an oral fentanyl lozenge that is available for treatment of your breakthrough pain when you are taking around-the-clock opioids.

Breakthrough pain can always occur even when you are taking your narcotic. Breakthrough pain means additional pain, which can occur when your activities increase. For example, if you go bowling you can have additional pain in addition to your usual chronic pain that must be treated.

Demerol (meperidine) is another drug that is available for pain management. It is not recommended for chronic pain because the break-down products of this drug can cause seizures and also because of its relatively short duration of pain-relieving action, one and a half to two hours, as compared to other opioid preparations.

Another drug called Ultram (tra-madol)is a weak narcotic-binding receptor drug that can decrease your pain. It also inhibits the reuptake of norepinephrine and serotonin, which are two chemicals that exist in your central nervous system that can also decrease your pain. If you are experiencing constipation, you should take a stool softener such as Colace.

If you develop nausea and vomiting associated with your narcotic medication, you may need a scopolamine skin patch. Another way of controlling your nausea and vomiting is with a rectal suppository of a medication that will stop your nausea and vomiting.

Clonidine (Catapress) may help control some cancer pains. The FDA has approved clonidine for epidural use. The epidural space is the spinal fluid that surrounds your spinal cord. Clonidine administered into your epidural space can control some pains that are caused by your cancer.

Narcotic medications can be placed into your epidural space or actually even placed into the fluid that surrounds your spinal cord through an implanted pump. A snail toxin called Prialt can also be placed in a pump to control your pain. This pump deposits the drug in the spinal fluid. Other routes of drug administration are the oral routes, but you do not have to swallow a pill.

Sublingual (under the tongue) morphine when it is in a high concentration (Roxanol 20 mg/ml) can provide you with pain relief if you cannot swallow pills. Actiq is a fentanyl preparation on a stick that resembles a lollipop.

Actiq works quickly to provide you with pain relief. An adhesive oral fentanyl disc is available which can control your pain as well. Rectal suppositories are another way of providing you with narcotic medications. Rectal suppositories are available for hydromorphone, oxymorphone, and morphine. The rectal administration of morphine, for example, can provide pain relief within 10 minutes.

Cancer pain can be successfully treated. In order to do so, a timely and accurate diagnosis must be done. This is one of many reasons why you should have a routine physical examination by your doctor.

Given that no two people are alike, if you are taking any medications and begin to take nutritional supplements you should be aware that potential drug-nutrient interactions may occur and are encouraged to consult a health care professional before using any natural product.

Combining certain prescription drugs and dietary supplements can lead to undesirable effects such as: diminished prescription drug effectiveness, reduced supplement effectiveness and impaired drug and/or supplement absorption.

Vitamin D, appears to have an effect on numerous disease states and disorders, including osteoporosis, chronic musculoskeletal pain, diabetes (types 1 and 2), multiple sclerosis, cardiovascular disease, and cancers of the breast, prostate, and colon.[1]

Relaxation may also be effective in treating the eating problems of the person with cancer, leading to improvement in weight and performance status.[2] Some human epidemiological studies on colon cancer point to a possible preventive role of dietary fiber, but the results are confounded by the difference in the intake of many other food substances such as fat and the overall differences in the dietary pattern of the populations investigated.[3]

Natural honey is a product with rich nutritional qualities that could be a pleasant, simple, and economic modality for the management of radiation mucositis.[4] A clove-based herbal mouthwash can have a potentially beneficial effect on minimizing or preventing radiation-induced oral mucositis in patients with head and neck cancer.[5]

It is shown how an unnaturally high omega-6/omega-3 fatty acid concentration ratio in meat, offal and eggs (because the omega-6/omega-3 ratio of the animal diet is unnaturally high) directly leads to exacerbation of pain conditions, cardiovascular disease and probably most cancers.[6]

References

1.      Grober U. [Vitamin D--an old vitamin in a new perspective]. Med Monatsschr Pharm. 2010;33(10):376-383.

2.      Campbell DF, Dixon JK, Sanderford LD, Denicola MA. Relaxation: its effect on the nutritional status and performance status of clients with cancer. J Am Diet Assoc. 1984;84(2):201-204.

3.       Spiller GA, Freeman HJ. Recent advances in dietary fiber and colorectal diseases. Am J Clin Nutr. 1981;34(6):1145-1152.

4.       Motallebnejad M, Akram S, Moghadamnia A, Moulana Z, Omidi S. The effect of topical application of pure honey on radiation-induced mucositis: a randomized clinical trial. J Contemp Dent Pract. 2008;9(3):40-47.

5.       Kong M, Hwang DS, Yoon SW, Kim J. The effect of clove-based herbal mouthwash on radiation-induced oral mucositis in patients with head and neck cancer: a single-blind randomized preliminary study. Onco Targets Ther. 2016;9:4533-4538.

6.       Christophersen OA, Haug A. Animal products, diseases and drugs: a plea for better integration between agricultural sciences, human nutrition and human pharmacology. Lipids Health Dis. 2011;10:16.

Vascular diseases have tendencies to obstruct blood flow to areas throughout your body. For example, patients with Raynaud's disease have complaints of burning pain, numbness and swelling in their fingers, toes or hands or feet on both arms. Raynaud's phenomenon usually involves one hand and is related to some lesion that compresses arteries to your hands. Raynaud's disease affects both hands while Raynaud's phenomenon can affect one hand.

Diseases that contribute to Raynaud's disease or phenomena include obstructive arterial disorders, vascular disorders, and scleroderma. Drug intoxications as well as some cancers and neurological entities can cause Raynaud's disease. Raynaud's disease is a vascular pain. Raynaud's disease pain can last a few minutes to hours. The average length of attack is 5 minutes to 60 minutes.

Raynaud's disease is a disorder of of blood flow to your fingers, toes, nose, ears, and sometimes your tongue. When you have symptoms, you will suddenly experience a decrease in your blood flow to these areas. You will have color changes of your skin, especially on your fingers and toes, with exposure to cold or emotional stress.

Cold exposure to your face can also cause changes in your fingers and toes. Many people use the term Raynaud's disease to include Raynaud's phenomena. This disease is classified as one of two types: primary and secondary. Secondary Raynaud's disease is also called Raynaud's phenomena.

Primary Raynaud's disease has no underlying medical problem and is mild and causes fewer complications than secondary Raynaud's disease.

Approximately 50 percent of people diagnosed with Raynaud's disease are primary Raynaud's disease and 50 percent are Raynaud's phenomena. Women are five times more likely than men to develop primary Raynaud's disease. Most patients develop Raynaud's disease before age 40.

Be aware that 30 percent of individuals with primary Raynaud's disease progress to secondary Raynaud's disease. Approximately 15 percent of individuals with primary Raynaud's disease do improve. The secondary Raynaud's disease or Raynaud's phenomena is essentially the same as primary Raynaud's disease but secondary Raynaud's disease occurs in individuals who have predisposing factors.

You need to know that there are three phases of Raynaud's disease. When you are first exposed to cold, your small arteries contract and your fingers, toes, ears, or the tip of your nose and tongue become pale and white. This observation occurs because you are deprived of blood. Remember if you have an increased blood flow to your tissues, the tissue will appear red. After your oxygen is deprived, your blood vessels will expand.

It is the veins that expand most. The veins carry blood that has minimal or no oxygen. This will give your blood a bluish tint. The area of the low-oxygen-carrying blood will appear blue.

The area also feels cold to touch. When your arteries begin to dilate, the blood flow is increased. Oxygen is increased and your tissue color will appear normal.

I have mentioned the associated diseases that you might have if you have secondary Raynaud's disease. Primary Raynaud's disease can be later classified as a secondary Raynaud's disease after a predisposing underlying disease has been diagnosed. This observation is seen in 30 percent of patients. A secondary type of Raynaud's disease is more complicated and severe.

This type of Raynaud's disease is more likely to worsen. Diseases that can predispose you to secondary Raynaud's disease include scleroderma, SLE, rheumatoid arthritis, and polio. For some reason, herniated discs and spinal cord tumors as well as cerebrovascular accidents and polio can progress to Raynaud's disease.

Vascular pain in general can be divided into three categories: Arterial pain, pain due to dysfunction of the capillaries in your tissue and pain related to pathology of your vei
ns. You can have obstruction of both your arteries and veins of your limbs. When this happens you have what is called Burger's disease. Swelling of the small arteries and veins in your extremities causes this disease. The painful symptoms that you note are a result again of decreased oxygen flow to your tissues.

When your blood supply to a part of your body is decreased, which happens in Burger's disease, your oxygen to your tissue is significantly decreased. You will develop pain in the calves of your legs. If the oxygen deficit is extremely low, your nerves to your legs will suffer injury.

This nerve injury will cause you pain as well as lack of oxygen to your extremity muscles. If your pain is severe, you may not experience relief with rest. If your tissues are deprived of oxygen for a long time, you can develop ulcerations in your skin and also develop gangrene.

Another problem with your blood vessels that can cause you to have pain is Takayasu's syndrome. This syndrome is due to inflammation or swelling of your small arteries of the upper part of your body, including your eyes. It occurs more in young girls as well as young women. More than 60 percent of individuals complain of weakness and fever as well as joint pain and pain in the upper extremities. When this pain occurs, you will soon develop the pain about the arteries that are inflamed. This disease can progress to even cause you to have angina pectoris. If this angina pectoris progresses, you may have a heart attack as well.

Temporal arteritis is another inflammation of the large arteries, especially around your temples. Inflammation of one or both of these arteries can cause you to have significant headaches. It can also involve other branches of your carotid artery. Temporal arteritis occurs usually if you are over 55 years of age. Temporal arteritis is more common in women than in men.

Occasionally if you have temporal arteritis you will have headaches that are occasionally unbearable. Your headache will begin over your involved arteries. As stated, the pain mostly begins about your temples. However, this disease can also affect your occipital arteries. These are the arteries that are toward the back of your head and approximate an area where the back of your skull meets your neck.

You may have tenderness to touch over the swollen and inflamed arteries. The areas around your inflamed arteries are extremely sensitive to firm touch. You may even have decreased blood flow to your jaw muscles. Therefore, when you chew you may have significant pain in your jaw muscles. Temporal arteritis can affect arteries in multiple locations throughout your body.

You may develop a flulike syndrome with generalized muscle pain as well as fever and weakness. The muscle pain can progress and involve your neck, shoulders, and pelvis as well as your legs. The arteries are usually affected on both sides of your body.

Erythemalgia is a syndrome that can affect both your arms and your legs. The temperature in your extremities will be elevated and you will have redness in either your arms or legs. Along with the change in color, you will have burning pain as well as tingling in your extremities. Sometimes you will experience swelling in your hands and feet.

Usually this disease affects your legs. However, it can also affect your arms. This entity is usually seen if you are exposed to an increased temperature. When you experience the pain, it can last for a few minutes up to hours. This type of pain in this syndrome can be associated with diabetes.

Sickle cell disease affects the arteries throughout your body. This pain can be severe. The sickling cells can stop blood flow to your blood vessels. As a result, you have generalized lack of oxygen to all of your tissues and have severe pain. Sickle cell disease is inherited.

Sickle cell disease is more prevalent in African Americans or individuals of Mediterrean decent. In Africa, the sickle cell gene gave advantage to individuals because it would resist infection caused by malaria. This is the reason why the disease is prevalent in populations of African descent. The deposition of sickled cells within your arteries decreases blood flow to your tissues. This causes a painful crisis to the majority of your organs.

If you have sickle cell disease and if you have a painful crisis, you will note the development of severe pain. The frequency of the pain occurs most in the third and fourth decades.

Cold and infection can induce you to have a sickle cell crisis. Furthermore, dehydration and alcohol consumption can cause you to have a crisis as well as exposure to low-oxygen tension. You can have pain in different parts of your body. Chest pain can occur. This is usually accompanied by a fever.

You back, legs, and stomach may also develop significant pain. If you have pain in your abdomen, this pain can mimic appendicitis. The sickle cell related pain can last from hours to even weeks. You can have a gradual or sudden onset of pain. You can have decreased blood flow to your bone. This will cause some tissue death in your bone. You can have pain in your joints as well as swelling. This pain is severe enough to cause you to experience depression.

The initial treatment of this disease is usually the administration of either steroids or nonsteroidal anti-inflammatory drugs. If your pain is severe, your doctor may prescribe narcotic medications until your crisis subsides. If you have infection as a cause of your sickle cell crisis, you may require antibiotics. Because of the depression associated with this entity, you may need to have a psychological evaluation as well as the administration of antidepressant drugs. Sometimes narcotic medications are necessary for pain control.

Scleroderma also affects your skin. By definition, it is called "hard skin." It is uncommon. Scleroderma is classified according to the degree of your skin thickening. Scleroderma is most common in adults. However, it can be seen in children.

The hallmarks of scleroderma are light skin and Raynaud's phenomena. Scleroderma is a generalized disorder of the small arteries as well as the connective tissue around your arteries. Not only can your gastrointestinal tract be affected but also your lungs, your heart, and your kidneys.

Most all patients who have scleroderma have Raynaud's disease. Patients with scleroderma can have pallor of the digits following cold exposure or emotional stress. Your fingers and toes can turn blue followed by redness in addition to burning pain and tingling.

You may develop gangrene and your fingers and toes may end up with an amputation. Swelling can be seen over your hands and feet. Over time, thinning of your skin can occur. The thinning of your skin is easily noted over joints. Usually scleroderma begins before age 40 and is more common in females. Approximately 80 percent of scleroderma patients are females.

Scleroderma can affect your kidneys and may cause you to have kidney failure. Scleroderma can also affect your heart and cause heart arrhythmias and palpations.. You may need an echocardiograph if you have chest pain.

This test can reveal some thickening around the outer wall of your heart. You will have muscle pain as well as joint pain if you have scleroderma. You will have stiffness in the morning. Systemic lupus erythematosus is a disease of unknown cause. It can also be associated with .

Systemic lupus erythematosus (SLE) is caused by your body's production of antibodies that injure the tissues of some of your organs in your body. The symptoms can come and go. You may have a rash develop on your face. However, SLE can be life threatening if it involves your internal organs. SLE can cause you to have failure of your kidneys or hemorrhage as well as a pulmonary disease.

Dermatomyositis is an inflammatory disease that can affect your muscles. You will have muscle pain and tenderness. A rash usually accompanies this disease. The rash occurs on your upper eyelids. You may have some swelling around your eyes as well. You can have redness about the knuckles of your fingers.

This disease can affect almost any organ system in your body. You can have involvement of the muscles of your fingers and toes. The muscles in your legs can become weak. This disease can be caused by an abnormality in your immune system. The diagnosis of this disease can be done by taking samples of your muscle.

Polyarteritis nodosa is caused by inflammation or swelling of the walls of your blood vessels. This disease can affect blood vessels of any size as well as in any location. It usually occurs between ages 40 and 50. Men are affected more than women. Your kidneys can be affected. If the disease progresses, you can develop kidney failure.

This disease can affect your arteries going to your heart and can cause you to have a heart attack. It may cause abdominal pain and bleeding. This disease can affect your nervous system as well. It can cause you to have weakness as well as loss of sensation. As stated previously, it can be associated with rheumatoid arthritis.

Given that no two people are alike, if you are taking any medications and begin to take nutritional supplements you should be aware that potential drug-nutrient interactions may occur and are encouraged to consult a health care professional before using any natural product.

Combining certain prescription drugs and dietary supplements can lead to undesirable effects such as: diminished prescription drug effectiveness, reduced supplement effectiveness and impaired drug and/or supplement absorption.

An increased dietary whole-grain intake may protect against cardiovascular disease in some individuals.[1]   Magnesium supplementation was reported to be associated with better blood pressure control, improved endothelial function and amelioration of subclinical atherosclerosis in some patients.[2]

The Mediterranean Diet is associated with a reduced incidence of vascular events[3] Omega 3 supplementation has been shown to improve large arterial elasticity and arterial blood pressure in some patients as well.[4] Acai consumption was reported to be associated with improvements in vascular function, which may lower the risk of a cardiovascular events as well.[5]

An eating pattern, characterized by high consumption of red and processed meat, alcohol, and sugar-sweetened beverages, and by frequent snacking and eating out as part of an overall unhealthy life-style, is associated with an increased prevalence, burden, and multisite presence of subclinical atherosclerosis.[6] This disease will cause vascular pain.

References

1.      Kirwan JP, Malin SK, Scelsi AR, et al. A Whole-Grain Diet Reduces Cardiovascular Risk Factors in Overweight and Obese Adults: A Randomized Controlled Trial. J Nutr. 2016;146(11):2244-2251.

2.      Cunha AR, D'El-Rei J, Medeiros F, et al. Oral magnesium supplementation improves endothelial function and attenuates subclinical atherosclerosis in thiazide-treated hypertensive women. J Hypertens. 2016.

3.      Pastori D, Carnevale R, Menichelli D, et al. Is There an Interplay Between Adherence to Mediterranean Diet, Antioxidant Status, and Vascular Disease in Atrial Fibrillation Patients? Antioxid Redox Signal. 2016;25(14):751-755.

4.      Chan DC, Pang J, Barrett PH, et al. Effect of omega-3 fatty acid supplementation on arterial elasticity in patients with familial hypercholesterolaemia on statin therapy. Nutr Metab Cardiovasc Dis. 2016.

5.          Alqurashi RM, Galante LA, Rowland IR, Spencer JP, Commane DM. Consumption of a flavonoid-rich acai meal is associated with acute improvements in vascular function and a reduction in total oxidative status in healthy overweight men. Am J Clin Nutr. 2016;104(5):1227-1235.

6.          Penalvo JL, Fernandez-Friera L, Lopez-Melgar B, et al. Association Between a Social-Business Eating Pattern and Early Asymptomatic Atherosclerosis. J Am Coll Cardiol. 2016;68(8):805-814.

# 34. CHEST PAIN

Chest pain is difficult to diagnose. Chest pain is vague. There are many structures in your chest cavity. You have two lungs, a diaphragm, a heart and a larynx and an esophagus. Furthermore, these organs have wrappers around them. The organs are wrapped by a peritoneum. The peritoneum contains many pain fibers. If your peritoneum becomes inflamed you may experience chest pain.

The heart's function is to pump blood. The right side of the heart pumps blood to the lungs, where oxygen is added to the blood and carbon dioxide is removed from it. The left side pumps blood to the rest of the body, where oxygen and nutrients are delivered to tissues and waste products are transferred to the blood for removal by other organs. The increase in heart size is mainly due to an increase in the size of

Because arteries and arterioles become less elastic as you get older, they cannot relax as quickly during the pumping of the heart. As a result, blood pressure increases in the older individual more when the heart contracts. High blood pressure during systole with normal blood pressure during diastole is very common among older people and this disorder is called isolated systolic hypertension.

Many of the effects of aging on the heart and blood vessels can be reduced by regular exercise. Exercise helps you maintain cardiovascular fitness as well as muscular fitness. Exercise is beneficial regardless of the age at which it is initiated.

The arteries can become clogged over time. If one of your arteries that supplies blood to your heart muscle is deprived of oxygen, you will experience chest pain (angina). If the lumen of your artery is completely obliterated then your heart muscle can become damaged causing you to have a heart attack (myocardial infarction). These changes occurred over time.

Angina is pain in the center of your chest. Usually rest relieves angina. Anginal chest pain in men may spread to the jaws and arms. Pain that radiates from the left side of the chest into the left arm is especially characteristic of anginal pain in men.

In women on the other hand, a decrease in oxygen to the heart muscle for some reason, causes anginal pain and pressure in the center of the chest accompanied by pain in the neck or arms. Angina or heart pain occurs when the demand for blood by the heart muscle exceeds the oxygen supply of the arteries. This why exercise like shoveling snow can cause angina.

A myocardial infarction (heart attack) or death of a segment of your heart muscle occurs following interruption of the blood supply to the heart muscle. This is more severe than angina. A heart attack can cause sudden severe chest pain. There is a danger that your heart could go into an irregular heartbeat called an arrhythmia.

If you have a severe arrhythmia, your heart can stop, which is referred to as a cardiac arrest. If you have interruption of the blood flow going to your heart, you can have irreversible injury to your heart muscle. This injury usually begins within 20 minutes from the time of the loss of blood flow to your heart muscle. Therefore, if you think that you are having a heart attack, contact your local emergency room or your doctor. If your pain is severe, go directly to your emergency room by ambulance.

Angina pectoris is chest pain that results from decreased oxygen supply to your heart muscle. Angina pectoris is usually pain under your breastbone. You may perceive discomfort instead of pain or pressure. The pain, if it is present or the pressure can radiate to your neck or arm that is usually your left arm.

Shortness of breath may also be reported. Angina pectoris is usually elicited by physical exertion. Occasionally psychological stress can cause you to have angina pectoris. If you are worried about an impending job interview for example, you could develop angina. Exposure to cold air can cause angina. Angina comes on quickly and can last for up to 15 minutes. It usually resolves with rest or with nitroglycerin.

Coronary artery disease can be a cause of angina. Over time coronary artery disease can also cause you to have a heart attack (myocardial infarction). Lifestyle changes such as diet, exercise, and stopping smoking tobacco can decrease the incidence of coronary artery disease. Atherosclerosis is a build-up of fat and other materials in the walls of arteries that causes them to become narrowed. This entity is caused by many factors. If you are hypertensive and have an elevated cholesterol and smoke, you are at a higher risk for developing atherosclerosis.

When you have a deposit of fat and calcium in your blood vessels, your heart will still pump blood through these vessels. It takes a decrease in the diameter of your blood vessels by approximately 70 percent to decrease your blood flow. Smoking is an important factor that can cause you to be at a high risk for developing coronary artery disease.

When you smoke tobacco, the nicotine in the tobacco causes your coronary arteries to decrease in caliber. This action decreases blood flow to your heart muscles that decreases oxygen to your heart muscles. A decreased in heart muscle oxygen can cause a heart attack.

A high cholesterol blood level can increase your risk of developing coronary artery disease. If you have high levels of low-density lipoprotein cholesterol, you have an elevated chance of developing coronary heart disease. If your cholesterol is elevated, your doctor will help you reduce your cholesterol with both diet and with pharmacologic management.

You must monitor your diet for fat intake. Cocaine can also contribute to heart disease. Cocaine use has become more and more prevalent in the United States. However, cocaine use can make the arteries in your heart to go into spasm. Cocaine can accelerate the deposition of fat and calcium in your blood vessels, which can cause you to have angina as well as a heart attack.

You will develop chest pain when your heart oxygen demand exceeds the supply of oxygen that your blood vessels are delivering to your heart. If your heart begins beating faster, the increase in oxygen demand is met by an increased blood flow in your arteries about your heart.

The small arteries around your heart muscle will increase their diameter to provide your heart with more oxygenated blood. If your vessels cannot dilate, your heart will not receive enough oxygen and you will experience pain in your chest. Fat and calcium within your heart vessels will restrict the amount of blood that goes to your heart.

According to the American Heart Association, approximately 6.3 million men and 6.6 million women in the United States have heart attacks. In the year 2000, more than 500,000 people died from heart disease. Different types of angina have been described.

Stable angina is angina that is chronic and is usually caused by physical activity or emotional stress. Stable angina is usually heart-related pain relieved by rest or nitroglycerin.

Unstable angina, on the other hand, can increase with rest. Other types of unstable angina can occur at low activity levels. Unstable angina may not be responsive to nitroglycerin. Sometimes you can develop spasms of your arteries that supply your heart muscle. This type of spasm is called Pinzmetal's angina and can be relieved frequently with nitroglycerin.

Stable angina is a term used to describe pain that is predictably caused by narrowing of your coronary arteries and a given stress to your heart. Shoveling the snow off your steps can cause you to experience angina. The pain is predictable in terms of its severity, how long it lasts, and what brings about relief (such as a single tablet of nitroglycerin placed under the tongue).

On the other hand, unstable angina describes a new pattern of pain not previously experienced, for example, pain previous-ly felt after a flight of stairs is now suddenly experienced at rest. Unstable angina is a medical emergency that should be immediately evaluated by a doctor.

In many instances during an angina attack your EKG, (a tracing of the electrical activity of your heart) may show signs of cardiac injury. However, it is also possible that your EKG can be completely normal, and this finding does not rule out heart attack or angina.

If you are having chest pain and your EKG appears normal, your doctor may do an echocardiogram or administer radioactive dye and do a heart perfusion study. Your doctor may take a sample of your blood to have it analyzed for any elevations of your heart enzymes.

If you have heart muscle damage, the injured tissue will release chemicals called isoenzymes. If these heart isoenzymes are increased, this may be a sign that you are having a heart attack. If you have a history of risk factors for coronary artery disease and if your symptoms are stable, your doctor may do a pharmacologic stress test.

A dobutamine echocardiogram study may be done. You will be given a drug that will increase your heart rate. You will be monitored with a continuous EKG to see if there are any changes on your EKG that suggest decreased perfusion to your heart muscles. Occasionally your cardiologist may want to do a coronary angiogram, which is a test that uses a dye to assess the extent of your coronary artery disease.

A chest pain syndrome that may be more prevalent in women is an entity called syndrome X. If you have this syndrome, you may have an exaggerated response of the small arteries that go to your heart muscles. This exaggerated response is constriction of the diameter of your arteries.

When this happens, you have decreased blood flow going to your heart. Usually women that suffer from this illness have a general-zed increase in their body pain overall. This disease is undergoing further research at present. The prevalence of the cardiac syndrome X is higher in women when compared to men. Estrogen deficiency has been shown to play a major role in the origin of cardiac syndrome X.

Aspirin can affect your blood's ability to clot and, if you are having angina or if you suspect that you are having a heart attack, aspirin can be lifesaving. Nutrients such as fish oils might be effective for the prevention of heart disease.

Remember that angina (heart pain) is not a heart attack. Angina is your body's warning to you that something is only means that some of your heart muscle is not getting enough blood temporarily.

A heart attack, on the other hand, occurs when the blood flow to your heart muscle is suddenly and permanently cut off. This event will usually cause permanent damage to your heart muscle. If you have angina, you must assume that you have underlying coronary artery disease unless proven otherwise.

If you have unstable angina or chest pain at rest, you may need hospitalization for intensive medical therapy. Aspirin and heparin can be given to decrease the clotting factors of your bloodstream. If you have angina, these drugs can decrease the progression of angina to a heart attack.

If you suspect that you are having a heart attack, seek immediate medical attention. Most deaths associated with an acute heart attack occur during the first hours following the onset of the heart attack. Nitroglycerine and morphine might be administered to you through your veins. If your heart rate is abnormal, your cardiologist will treat your abnormal heart rate as well.

Your EKG can be sent by telemetry by your emergency medical technician to a local emergency room so that the emergency room doctor can make a diagnosis of your heart rhythm and recommend any treatments that may be immediately necessary. It is important that blood is restored to your heart muscle. Sometimes your blood flow to your heart muscles can be increased by administering therapy to you that will break up blood clots in your heart blood vessels.

Streptokinase is one drug that can be used in this situation. You will be confined to bed for 24 to 36 hours. You will be placed in a cardiac care unit. Your activities will be gradually increased. There are enzymes that are released into your bloodstream when you have heart muscle damage.

Other medicines called as beta blockers can be used to slow your heart rate and decrease the contraction of your heart muscles. This maneuver will conserve oxygen.

Propranolol (Inderal) is an example of a beta blocker. Calcium channel blockers (Verapamil) affect the calcium in your muscle cells. Calcium channel blockers such as Verapamil can decrease the incidence of you having angina as well as a heart attack. If medication fails to control your angina, coronary artery bypass surgery is sometimes necessary.

A blood vessel is grafted onto your blocked artery. This allows your blood flow to bypass the blockage so that blood can go to your heart muscle to provide your heart muscle with needed oxygen. Your surgeon can use an artery inside your chest or take a vein from your leg.

Another treatment that can be used to increase your artery size is called balloon angioplasty. This involves insertion of a catheter that has a tiny balloon on the end of it into an artery either in your arm or your leg. The balloon is inflated briefly to widen your vessel in places where your arteries are narrow.

Another type of procedure that can increase your blood flow to your heart is called a stent. A stent is a surgical procedure, but it is a minor procedure compared to open-heart surgery. Stents are implanted through your veins with a catheter. The stent expands when it is placed. The stent will provide better blood flow at the location of your artery where the blood flow is decreased. The purpose of the stent is to permanently hold your artery open.

There are three other causes of non-cardiac chest pain that you should be familiar with; intercostal neuropathy, costochondritis and Tsetse's syndrome. Injury to your nerve under your rib bone can occur following a rib fracture, lung surgery or heart surgery or from an infection.

This pain may be relieved by anticonvulsant and/or antidepressant drugs. In some instances, your intercostal nerve needs to be injected with a local anesthetic with a steroid. If this fails, freezing the nerve with a cryo probe can provide you with significant pain relief.

Tietze's syndrome usually occurs in individuals less than 40 years of age. Usually only one pain site is experienced by this syndrome. It occurs at the junction between your ribs and your breast-bone (sternum) at the level of your second rib.

Costochondritis usually occurs in individuals over 40. More than one area of pain is involved and is at the levels of your second to fifth ribs. Tietze's syndrome follows a respiratory infection while costochondritis follows a neck sprain or coronary heart disease. The treatment of these two pain syndromes is the same as the intercostal neuropathy with the exception that injection therapy is done at the location of the pain.

Given that no two people are alike, if you are taking any medications and begin to take nutritional supplements you should be aware that potential drug-nutrient interactions may occur and are encouraged to consult a health care professional before using any natural product.

Combining certain prescription drugs and dietary supplements can lead to undesirable effects such as: diminished prescription drug effectiveness, reduced supplement effectiveness and impaired drug and/or supplement absorption.

Some prospective studies showed a direct inverse association between fruit and vegetable intake and the development of cardio vascular disease (CVD) incidents such as acute plaque rupture causing unstable angina or myocardial infarction and stroke.

Many nutrients and phytochemicals in fruits and vegetables, including fiber, potassium, and folate, could be independently or jointly responsible for the apparent reduction in CVD risk. Novel findings and critical appraisal regarding antioxidants, dietary fibers, omega-3 polyunsaturated fatty acids), nutraceuticals, vitamins, and minerals.[1]

High red meat intake increases risk of coronary artery disease and that coronary heart disease (CHD) risk may be reduced importantly by shifting sources of protein in the US diet.

Exclusive use of olive oil during food preparation seems to offer significant protection against CHD, irrespective of various clinical, lifestyle and other characteristics of the participants.[2] Flaxseed is also an important source of alpha-linolenic acid an essential omega-3 fatty acid.[3]

Current recommendations to reduce cardiovascular risk include maintaining a healthy body weight, eating five or more portions of fruit and vegetables each day, reducing intake of fat (particularly saturated fatty acids), reducing salt intake and eating one portion of oily fish per week.[4] The Mediterranean diet adherence was associated with a significantly reduced CHD risk

References

1.       Ignarro LJ, Balestrieri ML, Napoli C. Nutrition, physical activity, and cardiovascular disease: an update. Cardiovasc Res. 2007;73(2):326-340.

2.       Kontogianni MD, Panagiotakos DB, Chrysohoou C, Pitsavos C, Zampelas A, Stefanadis C. The impact of olive oil consumption pattern on the risk of acute coronary syndromes: The CARDIO2000 case-control study. Clin Cardiol. 2007;30(3):125-129.

3.       Leyva DR, Zahradka P, Ramjiawan B, Guzman R, Aliani M, Pierce GN. The effect of dietary flaxseed on improving symptoms of cardiovascular disease in patients with peripheral artery disease: rationale and design of the FLAX-PAD randomized controlled trial. Contemp Clin Trials. 2011;32(5):724-730.

4.       Kelly CN, Stanner SA. Diet and cardiovascular disease in the UK: are the messages getting across? Proc Nutr Soc. 2003;62(3):583-589.

Pain in your abdomen bladder and kidney can be disabling and severe. Abdominal pain in general occurs more often in women than in men. Stress, diet, and the work environment may be causes of abdominal pain in general. Cramping and intermittent pain is easily caused by disorders of your bowel, gallbladder, and ureter of your kidney or your fallopian tubes from your uterus.

Pain in your abdomen and pelvis is called visceral pain and is non-specific with respect to the exact location of your pain. Many nerves from many organs can send pain signals to your spinal cord and brain.

A common syndrome in adults is the irritable bowel syndrome (IBS), which is frequently diagnosed in the general population. Approximately 30 percent of patients seen by gastroenterologists suffer from IBS. It is more common in women and may even be seen in adolescents. If you have IBS, this disease can impair your quality of life.

The exact cause of IBS remains to be discovered. IBS can be caused by physiological, psychological, and behavioral factors. Sometimes you may have severe symptoms without any physical findings. This pain is not confined to one area of your gut but it is global over your stomach. Sometimes IBS is diagnosed in patients who suffer from fibromyalgia.

Usually this abdominal pain associated with IBS is relieved followed a bowel movement. You may suffer diarrhea alternating with constipation. You may have bloating or the feeling of incomplete evacuation of your stool following a bowel movement.

Some physicians believe that your colon is the cause of IBS. You can have symptoms daily or you may have symptoms once a week or once a month. If you have IBS, you may also have heartburn and nausea. IBS is sometimes associated with fibromyalgia. You may also suffer from chronic fatigue and significant depression.

Pain associated with IBS can be caused by depression or other behav-ioral illnesses. If you have psychosocial factors, these factors can influ-ence the frequency of your symptoms as well as the severity of your symptoms. If you suffer from IBS, you may have a previous history of physical, sexual, or emotional abuse.

To be diagnosed with IBS, you need to have abdominal pain first of all. Your pain must be relieved with a bowel movement. The onset of your pain must be associated with a change in the frequency of your stool habits.

The onset of your pain must be associated with a change in the appearance of your stool. If you have bloating or abdominal distention in one out of four days or passage of mucus in one out of four defecations, there is a high probability that you have IBS.

It is now accepted that if you suffer from IBS, you are not "crazy." It is known through recent research that nerves in your gastrointestinal system can become oversensitive, causing them to overreact to both gas as well as food passing by these nerves. The stimulation of your nerves in your gastro-intestinal tract will cause you to have pain as well as cramping.

If you have moderate symptoms, you may require psychological treatment and occasionally pharmacologic management. If you have severe and constant symptoms, you may require antidepressants as well as psycho-logical testing and treatment and you may need to be referred to a specialist in abdominal diseases (gastroenterologist).

The possibility of developing IBS is extremely high in individuals who suffer panic disorders. If you have moderate to severe depression, you are also prone to IBS. The reason for this association remains unknown.

Your brain can affect the nerves in your stomach and cause you to have an upset stomach. For example, if you are anxious or have to give a speech in front of a large crowd, you may develop "butterflies" in your stomach. You might feel the effect of your stress within your gastrointestinal system.

The newer drug Lotronex (alosetron) is used to treat abdominal pain and discomfort as well as any symptoms of diarrhea. Lotronex is the first drug approved by the FDA to be used for IBS treatment. Another newer drug designed to treat IBS that is now unavailable is called Zelnorm (tegaser-od).

It is a drug that is in a class of medications called gastrointestinal ser-otonin agonists. This drug is used for the treatment of constipation, bloating, and abdominal pain. Because of serious side effects this drug was withdrawn from the market in March 2007. If you suffer from IBS, you may want to minimize your fat intake.

Gastro esophageal reflux disease (GERD) can cause burning pain in your lower thorax or your upper abdomen. It is caused by relaxation of the lower esophageal sphincter that allow stomach acid to go into your esopha-gus. This condition can be treated with ant acids. Upper abdominal pain can come from a hiatal hernia. You may have vomiting as well as generalized abdominal pain. In this condition, your stomach herniates into your chest cavity. You may require surgery to correct this deformity.

Abdominal pain can come from ulcers where the lining of your stomach or duodenum is injured or you may have gastritis where the lining of your stomach is inflamed. Treatment for ulcers and gastritis include antacids, H2 blockers like cimetidine and if no relief occurs with these medications the use of protein pump inhibitors like omeprazole (Zegerid) may be therapeutic.

Your pancreas can also be a source of severe pain. The pain in acute situations can radiate from your mid abdomen to your back. Alcohol or a gallstone can injure your pancreas. A lab test that measures your blood amylase level will be abnormal if you have acute pancreatitis. An ultra sound will help in the diagnosis of pancreatic disease. You will need fluid replacement and analgesic medications such as narcotics if you have an acute attack of pancreatitis.

Chronic pancreatitis is an inflammation seen usually in chronic alcoholics. The diagnosis is made with a CAT scan or ultrasound or an endoscopic retrograde cholangio pancrea tography (ERCP). To help with chronic pain you may need destruction of the nerves going to your pancreas called the celiac plexus. This injection can be done with alcohol or phenol.

An appendix or gallbladder inflammation can also be very painful. Your gallbladder is in the upper right side of your abdomen while your appendix is located in the right lower aspect of your abdomen. If either of these organs becomes diseased, you can develop nausea, vomiting and a fever. Surgery may be necessary to remove one of these diseased organs. Laboratory tests, antibiotics and analgesics are necessary.

A CAT scan or a HIDA study can be used to diagnose gallbladder disease. Approximately 20 % of patients continue to experience pain post gallbladder surgery. The reason is usually related to a gallstone in the common bile duct. Appendicitis can be diagnosed with an abdominal ultrasound in most cases.

Your immune system can be a cause of abdominal pain. Inflammatory bowel disease is believed to be a disease of your immune system. IBS can respond to diet. However, the inflammatory bowel disease rarely responds to changes in diet. Inflammatory bowel disease includes ulcerative colitis and Crohn's disease. Ulcerative colitis is a chronic disease and a recurrent disease. It involves inflammation of the lining of the colon. It can also involve your rectum.

Crohn's disease can involve any part of your gastrointestinal tract, including your mouth all the way to your anus. The causes of Crohn's disease and ulcerative colitis are unknown. Usually inflammatory bowel disease begins in early adult life. However, there are cases reported in the elderly.

Genetic factors can make you prone to inflammatory bowel disease. If you have a disorder of your immune system, you are again prone to develop irritable bowel disease. It is possible that your immune system may attack the lining of your gastrointestinal system.

Crohn's disease involves the lower ileum (the lowest part of the small intestine). Your rectum can be involved as well. Approximately one third of Crohn's disease patients have their pathology in their colon, whereas one third of patients have their pathology in their ileum and one third have their pathology in both their ileum and colon. The inflammation of your gastrointestinal system can go from the inside of your bowel to the outside.

The inner lining of your gastrointestinal tract can develop ulcers in some cases of Crohn's disease. An ulcer is a break in the lining of the wall of your stomach or small intestine. This break in your gut lining can fail to heal and can be accompanied by inflammation. A fistula from the inside of your bowel to the outside can develop. A fistula is an abnormal communication between a hollow organ and the exterior.

If you have Crohn's disease, you can have an increased incidence of gallstones. With Crohn's disease, your bile salts may not be absorbed properly through your ileum. You can also develop kidney stones. You can have a history of frequent liquid bowel movements.

Because of absorption problems of nutrients, you may have a poor nutritional status. You can feel fatigued and suffer from a loss of energy. This thickened loop of inflamed bowel can be tender to deep palpation. If you develop a tract from the inside of your bowel to the outside, this fistula can cause you to develop an abscess behind the lining of your bowel. You will have fever, chills, and tenderness to deep palpation about your abdomen.

A barium enema is an enema with opaque contrast liquid that outlines your intestines on x-ray images. This test helps your doctor look for abnormalities in your bowel.

To examine your lower bowel, your doctor may also use air with the barium to distend your bowel. Through the colonoscope (a flexible fiberoptic instrument), your physician can obtain biopsies of your colon and ilium. If your gastrointestinal system develops an obstruction somewhere in your system, your food cannot pass through this obstruction.

You will be treated with fluids through your veins, and a tube will be placed through your nose to suction out substances that are unable to pass through your bowel. Steroids can be necessary to treat the inflammation caused by Crohn's disease. Be aware that chronic cramping, abdominal pain, and diarrhea are noted in both IBS and Crohn's disease.

Antibiotics may be used for the treatment of an inflammatory disease. Sulfasalazine is effective in reducing the symptoms of your disease. Drugs that can affect your immune system such as azathioprine and mercaptopurine are also useful in the treatment of your disease if it is unresponsive to the other methods that we mentioned. If you smoke, stop smoking; smoking can cause you to have a recurrence of Crohn's symptoms. If conservative treatments fail, you may require surgery.

Ulcerative colitis is another form of inflammatory bowel disease. Ulcerative colitis involves an inflammation of the inner lining of your colon. You will have bloody diarrhea if you have ulcerative colitis. You will have pain in your abdomen. You can develop anemia and the protein in your bloodstream, albumin, will be decreased. A scope in your colon is the key to the diagnosis of your disease.

A hernia can cause abdominal pain. A hernia is an abnormal protrusion, or bulging out, of part of an organ such as a portion of your intestine through the tissues that normally contain it. In this condition, a weak spot or opening in a body wall, often due to laxity of the muscles, allows part of the organ to protrude causing a hernia to occur. A hernia may develop in almost any part of the body; but the muscles of the abdominal wall are most commonly affected.

Hernias cause pain and reduce general mobility. One major danger of a hernia is that if bowel is contained within the protruding loop it may hinder or stop the blood flow through the intestine (occlusion). More serious still, if the loop itself becomes twisted outside its containing structure, or compressed at the point where it breaks through that structure (a strangulated hernia), the blood supply to the loop will also cease and the entire hernia will undergo tissue death (necrosis). This requires immediate emergency surgery.

Although there are many types of hernias, the following are the most common: An abdominal hernia is also called an epigastric or ventral hernia. This type of hernia affects one person in 100.

This group of hernias also includes inguinal hernias and umbilical hernias. Indirect inguinal hernias affect men only. A loop of intestine passes down the canal from where a testis descends early in childhood into the scrotum. If neglected, this type of hernia tends to increase progressively in size causing the scrotum to expand.

On the other hand a direct inguinal hernia affects both sexes. The intestinal loop forms a swelling in the inner part of the fold of the groin. A femoral hernia also affects both sexes although most often women. An intestinal loop passes down the canal containing the major blood vessels to and from the leg, between the abdomen and the thigh, causing a bulge in the groin and another at the top of the inner thigh.

An umbilical hernia affects both sexes as well. An intestinal loop protrudes through a weakness in the abdominal wall at the navel. A hiatal hernia also affects both sexes. A loop of the stomach when particularly full protrudes upward through the small opening in the diaphragm through which the esophagus passes, thus leaving the abdominal cavity and entering the chest. An incisional hernia is a hernia that occurs at the site of a surgical incision. This is due to strain on the healing tissues due to excessive muscular effort, lifting, coughing, or extreme pressure.

An obturator hernia is a rare type of hernia, but it is a significant cause of intestinal obstruction due to the associated anatomy. This hernia can occur in your upper thigh. A correct diagnosis and treatment of an obturator hernia is important, because delay can lead to high mortality.

Umbilical hernias can be present from birth, but most happen later due to pressure on openings or weaknesses in the abdominal cavity or wall from heavy lifting etc. Hernias tend to run in families, and can be caused by such things as coughing, straining during a bowel movement, lifting heavy objects, accumulation of fluid in the abdominal cavity, and obesity.

The symptoms of hernias vary, depending on the cause and the structures involved. Most begin as small, hardly noticeable breakthroughs. At first, they may be soft lumps under the skin, a little larger than a marble; there usually is no pain. Gradually, the pressure of the internal contents against the weak wall increases, and the size of the lump increases.

Early on, the hernia may be reduced which means that the protruding structures can be pushed back into their normal places. If those structures, however, cannot be returned to their normal locations through manipulation, the hernia is said to be irreducible, or incarcerated. The treatment of an incarcerated abdominal hernia is a serious surgical problem. Operations may be marked by high mortality due to the late diagnosis of incarceration and further postoperative complications.

For small, non-strangulated and non-incarcerated hernias, various supports and trusses may offer temporary, symptomatic relief. However, the best treatment is surgical closure or repair of the muscle wall through which the hernia protrudes.

When the weakened area is very large, some strong synthetic material may be sewn over the defect to reinforce the weak area. Postoperative care involves protecting the patient from respiratory infections that might cause coughing or sneezing, which would strain the suture line. Recovery is usually quick and complete.

Be aware that pilonidal sinus disease is a common problem of the sacro coccygeal region. However, it is also observed in the periumbilical area. It is recommend that conservative treatment be done in patients an with umbilical pilonidal sinus. Surgery should be performed in recurrent cases resistant to conservative treatment. The importance of differential diagnosis of umbilical pilonidal sinus from other umbilical pathologies is emphasized.

Laparoscopic onlay patch hernioplasty is a safe and efficacious technique for the repair of umbilical hernia. Compared to the Mayo repair, the Laparoscopic approach confers the advantages of reduced postoperative pain, shorter hospital stay, and a diminished morbidity rate. It has been recommended that a surgeon use alloplastic material for umbilical hernia repair for patients with a BMI greater than 30.0 and hernia orifice larger than 3 cm.

The decision for use of a mesh in hernial gaps from 2 to 3 cm should depend on individual factors. Older age, severe coexisting diseases, and late hospitalization were the main causes of unfavorable outcomes of the management of incarcerated hernias.

Be aware also that compared with patients with aorto iliac occlusive disease, patients with an abdominal aortic aneurysm have a higher frequency of abdominal wall hernia and inguinal hernia, and are at significant increased risk for development of incision hernia postoperatively.

The higher frequency of hernia formation in patients with abdominal aoritic aneurysms suggests the presence of a structural defect within the fascia. Further studies are needed to delineate the molecular changes of the aorta and its relation to the abdominal wall fascia.

Patients who have had placement of a mesh graft can have lingering severe pain that may become disabling. Chronic inguinodynia or neuralgia after conventional inguinal herniorrhaphy is rare, and diagnosing the exact cause is difficult. Treatment has ranged from local injection to remedial surgery with variable results. The increasing popularity of prosthetic mesh repairs has not eliminated these pain syndromes from occasionally occurring.

It appears that coincident neurectomy affords better results than mesh removal alone. Despite the popularity and favorable outcomes of prosthetic mesh repairs, persistent postoperative pain still occurs in a small number of patients. This may become more evident with the rising interest in laparoscopy.

Female diseases may also cause abdominal pain. Endometriosis is a common and painful disorder in women where tissue that normally lines the inside of the uterus (the endometrium) becomes implanted on tissue outside the uterus such as the abdomen. This can cause women to have pain in their abdomen. However, organs that are part of your gastrointestinal system are usually the cause of your abdominal pain.

If you have pain in your upper abdomen on the right side, you may have an inflamed gallbladder or an ulcer. Hepatitis can cause you to have pain. Pancreatitis, a painful inflammation of the pancreas, can cause pain in your mid abdomen that radiates to your back.

Renal stones and kidney stones on occasion can cause abdominal pain in addition to pain in your flanks. Kidney pain can arise from increased pressure in your kidney capsule or in your ureter. Pain you're your ureter can be referred to your sides (flanks) or to your groin. If your kidney is inflamed as from a stone or infection, a punch over the area of your kidney can cause pain. If you have blood in your urine, you may have a stone.

If you are a male and if your scrotum is painful and swollen, you need to see your doctor, as you may have twisting of your spermatic cord or torsion of your spermatic cord. You may need surgery. If your scrotum is infected, it is called an epididymitis. Interstitial cystitis is an inflammatory disease of your bladder that can cause you to have lower abdominal pain.

If your abdominal pain is associated with your menstrual cycle, keep a diary of how the pain is affected. Ovarian cysts can cause you to have pain in your lower abdomen. Abdominal pain is the pain that you feel in your abdominal area that is between your chest and groin. Another term for abdomen is your stomach or "belly." Always be aware that pain in your abdomen can originate from your chest or your pelvis (the area below your abdomen).

Interstitial cystitis is a painful pelvic pain from the bladder with a cause that is unknown. An examination using a cystoscope by an urologist may reveal ulcerations in the lining of your bladder. The exact cause may be your immune system. Many treatments have been proposed including surgery on your bladder. Psychological treatment may help as well as installation of various substances into your bladder.

Blood vessels in your abdomen may also be a source of abdominal pain. For example, your aorta, which is a major blood vessel that comes off your heart, runs down through your abdomen and divides into major arteries that supply blood flow to your legs.

If you have an aneurysm, which is a defect in the wall of this great vessel, you can have pain in your abdomen. An aneurysm needs to be evaluated by your doctor.

An aneurysm is a weakness in the wall of your aorta. If you have abdominal pain and are able to feel or palpate a strong pulse in your abdomen you should consult with your physician. This weak area could rupture, which could be fatal. If you can feel a palpable mass in your abdomen this may be an aneurysm.  Ask your doctor if the mass that you feel is abnormal.

Your appendix, if it is inflamed, can cause you to have abdominal pain as well. Your appendix is part of your gastrointestinal system. If you have appendicitis, you will have pain in the right lower part of your abdomen.  You will experience nausea and vomiting and may have a fever.  It is important for you to see a doctor because an untreated appendicitis can rupture and cause peritonitis.  Peritonitis can be fatal.

A viral infection in your intestine or gas in your intestine can cause you to have significant abdominal pain. As you probably know, this pain can be severe. This should alert you that the severity of the pain does not correlate with the severity of the disease.

In other words, you can have cancer of your colon and have only mild pain. Causes of abdominal pain include gas, constipation, milk intolerance, stomach flu, an irritable bowel syndrome, indigestion, esophageal reflux, ulcers, gallstones, and diverticular disease.

Microorganisms can also be sources of abdominal pain. Parasites as well as bacteria like Helicobacter pylori can cause you to have abdominal pain. This bacterium is called in microbiological terms a gram-negative bacterium and can be found in the moist membrane lining of your stomach.

It can cause you to develop a progressive gastritis (an inflammation of the lining of your stomach) as well as stomach cancer, heart disease, and gastric and duodenal ulcers. Antibiotic therapy will be effective. If your pain is severe, you may require narcotics for your pain management.

Given that no two people are alike, if you are taking any medications and begin to take nutritional supplements you should be aware that potential drug-nutrient interactions may occur and are encouraged to consult a health care professional before using any natural product. Combining certain prescription drugs and dietary supplements can lead to undesirable effects such as: diminished prescription drug effectiveness, reduced supplement effectiveness and impaired drug and/or supplement absorption.

Dietary advice is considered to be of importance to reduce gastrointestinal (GI) symptoms in patients with diabetic gastroparesis. A small particle diet improves the key symptoms of gastroparesis in patients with diabetes mellitus.[1] Preliminary studies suggest low doses of prebiotics may improve symptoms of IBS, although further robust clinical trials are required.[2,3]

L-arginine can positively impact intestinal mucositis by promoting partial mucosal recovery, reducing inflammation and improving intestinal permeability.[4]

Kaempferol (KF) is the most abundant polyphenol in tea, fruits, vegetables, and beans. Kaempferol was shown to attenuate the expansion of inflammatory lesions seen in ethanol and aspirin-induced gastritis, pancreatitis, and acetic acid-induced writhing.[5]

Combination of early enteral nutrition and rhubarb significantly improved the gastrointestinal function, inhibited systemic inflammation and disease severity and mitigated the disease-related damages of liver and kidney function in acute pancreatitis patients.[6]

References

1.      Olausson EA, Storsrud S, Grundin H, Isaksson M, Attvall S, Simren M. A small particle size diet reduces upper gastrointestinal symptoms in patients with diabetic gastroparesis: a randomized controlled trial. Am J Gastroenterol. 2014;109(3):375-385.

2.      Whelan K. Probiotics and prebiotics in the management of irritable bowel syndrome: a review of recent clinical trials and systematic reviews. Curr Opin Clin Nutr Metab Care. 2011;14(6):581-587.

3.      Korpela R, Niittynen L. Probiotics and irritable bowel syndrome. Microb Ecol Health Dis. 2012;23.

4.      Leocadio PC, Antunes MM, Teixeira LG, et al. L-arginine pretreatment reduces intestinal mucositis as induced by 5-FU in mice. Nutr Cancer. 2015;67(3):486-493.

5.      Kim SH, Park JG, Sung GH, et al. Kaempferol, a dietary flavonoid, ameliorates acute inflammatory and nociceptive symptoms in gastritis, pancreatitis, and abdominal pain. Mol Nutr Food Res. 2015;59(7):1400-1405.

6.      Wan B, Fu H, Yin J, Xu F. Efficacy of rhubarb combined with early enteral nutrition for the treatment of severe acute pancreatitis: a randomized controlled trial. Scand J Gastroenterol. 2014;49(11):1375-1384.

Psychological illness can be associated with pain manifestations. The most common personality disorders are the somatoform disorders. The somatoform disorders are a group of mental disturbances that are diagnosed on the basis of their symptoms. These disorders are characterized by physical complaints that appear to be medical in origin but that cannot be explained in terms of a physical disease.

The physical symptoms must be serious enough to interfere with a patient's employment or relationships, and must not be under the patient's voluntary control in order to qualify as a somatoform disorder. In general, the somatoform disorders are characterized by disturbances in the patient's physical sensations or ability to move the limbs or walk, while the dissociative disorders are marked by disturbances in the patient's sense of identity or memory.

The physical symptoms are not under the patient's conscious control, so that he or she is not intentionally trying to confuse the doctor or complicate the process of diagnosis. Somatoform disorders are a significant problem for the health care system because these patients overuse medical services and resources.

A somatoform disorder that can be difficult to treat is the somatization disorder. The somatization disorder was formerly called Briquet's syndrome, after the French physician who first recognized it. The distinguishing characteristic of this disorder is a group or pattern of symptoms in several different organ systems of the patient's body that cannot be ascertained by a medical illness.

The diagnosis of the somatization disorder requires four symptoms of pain, two symptoms in the digestive tract, one symptom involving the sexual organs, and one symptom related to the nervous system.

The somatization disorder usually begins before the age of 30. It is estimated that 0.2% of the United States population will develop this disorder in the course of their lives. The female-to-male ratio is estimated to range between 5:1 and 20:1.

The somatization disorder is considered a chronic disturbance that tends to persist throughout the patient's life. It usually begins in the teenage years. It is also likely to run in families. A conversion disorder may be suspected in individuals who experience a loss of sensation without a medical cause.

A conversion disorder is a condition in which the patient's senses or ability to walk or move are impaired without a recognized medical or neurological disease or cause and in which psychological factors such as stress or trauma are the causes of this disorder.

In this disorder, the patient is converting a psychological conflict or problem into an inability to move specific parts of the body or to use the senses normally.

A conversion reaction contains the anxiety and serves to get the patient out of the threatening situation. The resolution of the emotion that underlies the physical symptom is called the patient's primary gain, and the change in the patient's social, occupational, or family situation that results from the symptom is called a secondary gain.

Some physical symptoms of a conversion disorder include a loss of balance, paralysis of an arm or leg, the inability to swallow or speak; the loss of touch or pain sensation; loss of sight or hearing, double vision or having seizures.

Unlike the somatization disorder, a conversion disorder may begin at any age, and it does not appear to run in families. A conversion disorder usually occurs among less educated or sophisticated people. A conversion disorder is not usually a chronic disturbance. The female-to-male ratio is 2:1. Male patients are likely to develop conversion disorders in occupational settings or military service.

Another personality disorder is the pain disorder. The pain disorder is noted by the presence of severe pain as the patient's focus. This category of somatoform disorder covers a range of patients with a variety of ailments, including chronic headaches, back problems, arthritis, muscle aches and cramps, or pelvic pain.

In some cases the patient's pain appears to be largely due to psychological factors, but in other cases the pain is derived from a medical condition as well as the patient's psychology. This disorder is seen in older patients.

Hypochondriasis is a somatoform disorder marked by excessive fear of or preoccupation with having a serious illness that persists in spite of negative medical testing. Hypochondriasis is usually seen in young adults. Flare-ups of this disorder are often correlated with stressful events in the patient's life.

Both the somatization disorder and hypochondriasis may result from the patient's unconscious reflection or imitation of parental behaviors. This behavior is particularly likely if the patient's parent derived considerable secondary gain from his or her symptoms.

An accurate diagnosis of somatoform disorders is important to prevent unnecessary pain procedures, surgery, laboratory tests, or other treatments and procedures. The diagnosis of somatoform disorders requires a thorough physical workup to exclude medical and neurological conditions as a cause of a pain disorder. A detailed examination is necessary when conversion disorder is a possible diagnosis.

In addition to anxiety or, the doctor must consider major depression as a possible additional diagnosis when evaluating a patient with symptoms of a somatoform disorder. Because patients with somatoform disorders often have lengthy medical histories, a long-term relationship with a primary care practitioner can prevent unnecessary treatments by specialists to a minimum.

Patients with somatoform disorders may be treated with antianxiety drugs or antidepressant drugs. The treatment should be directed to symptom reduction and stabilization of the patient's personality.

Another psychological disorder seen in the pain patient population is the factitious disorder. Factitious disorders are a group of mental disturbances in which patients intentionally act physically or mentally ill without obvious benefits. The name factitious comes from a Latin word that means artificial. These disorders are not malingering.

Patients with factitious disorders exaggerate the symptoms of a physical or mental illness by a variety of methods, including contaminating urine samples with blood, taking hallucinogens or injecting themselves with bacteria. These disorders are more common in men than in women.

The Munchausen syndrome refers to patients whose factitious symptoms are dramatized and exaggerated. Many persons with Munchausen undergo major surgery repeatedly. These patients have a pathological desire to be sick.

Patients with somatoform disorders believe that they have a physical disease. Malingering on the other hand is a deliberate behavior for a known external purpose. It is not considered a form of mental illness or psychopathology. A malinger may have valid symptoms but is dishonest as to the source of the problems. The individual may have sustained a disc herniation from a fall at home but claimed that it happened at work to be able to get compensation.

An injury that resulted from an automobile accident may be exaggerated for financial gain. Examples include months of chiropractic treatment for low back pain, or physical therapy without improvement.

This is not to be confused with those patients who have legitimate serious injuries that fail to respond to conservative treatment. There is usually a marked discrepancy between the person's claimed symptoms and the medical findings in a malingerer.

Given that no two people are alike, if you are taking any medications and begin to take nutritional supplements you should be aware that potential drug-nutrient interactions may occur and are encouraged to consult a health care professional before using any natural product.

Combining certain prescription drugs and dietary supplements can lead to undesirable effects such as: diminished prescription drug effectiveness, reduced supplement effectiveness and impaired drug and/or supplement absorption.

Hypovitaminosis C and D are highly prevalent in acutely hospitalized patients, but the clinical significance of these biochemical abnormalities is not known. Because deficiencies of vitamin C and D have been linked to psychologic abnormalities, vitamin C or D provision could improve the mood state of acutely hospitalized patients. Treatment of hypovitaminosis C improves the mood state of acutely hospitalized patients.[1]

Omega-3 and omega-6 fatty acids are precursors of bioactive lipid mediators posited to modulate both physical pain and psychological distress. Dietary manipulation of n-3 and n-6 fatty acids, previously shown to produce major improvements in headache, was found to also reduce psychological distress.[2]

It has been proposed that the association between life stress, physiologic response and chronic conditions is modified by nutritional status, with a focus on B vitamins and antioxidant vitamins.[3]

Stress, malnutrition and physical inactivity are three maternal behavioral lifestyle factors that can influence immune and central nervous system functions in both the mother and fetus, and may therefore, increase risk for neurodevelopmental/psychiatric disorders.[4]

A substantial proportion of noncommunicable disease originates in habitual overconsumption of calories, which can lead to weight gain and obesity and attendant comorbidities. At the other end of the spectrum, the consequences of undernutrition in early life and at different stages of adult life can also have major impact on wellbeing and quality of life.

To help address some of these issues, greater understanding is required of interactions with food and contemporary diets throughout the life course and at a number of different levels: physiological, metabolic, psychological, and emotional.[5]

There is support for the efficacy of omega-3, vitamin, and mineral supplementation in reducing aggressive behavior in children, and represent the first evaluation of nutritional supplements in conjunction with cognitive behavioral therapy.[6]

It is increasingly appreciated that perinatal events can set an organism on a life-long trajectory for either health or disease, resilience or risk. One early life variable that has proven critical for optimal development is the nutritional environment in which the organism develops. Extensive research has documented the effects of both undernutrition and over nutrition, with strong links evident for an increased risk for obesity and metabolic disorders, as well as adverse mental health outcomes.[7]

References

1.      Zhang M, Robitaille L, Eintracht S, Hoffer LJ. Vitamin C provision improves mood in acutely hospitalized patients. Nutrition. 2011;27(5):530-533.

2.      Ramsden CE, Faurot KR, Zamora D, et al. Targeted alterations in dietary n-3 and n-6 fatty acids improve life functioning and reduce psychological distress among patients with chronic headache: a secondary analysis of a randomized trial. Pain. 2015;156(4):587-596.

3.      Tucker KL. Stress and nutrition in relation to excess development of chronic disease in Puerto Rican adults living in the Northeastern USA. J Med Invest. 2005;52 Suppl:252-258.

4.      Marques AH, Bjorke-Monsen AL, Teixeira AL, Silverman MN. Maternal stress, nutrition and physical activity: Impact on immune function, CNS development and psychopathology. Brain Res. 2015;1617:28-46.

5.      Murphy M, Mercer JG. Diet-regulated anxiety. Int J Endocrinol. 2013;2013:701967.

6.      Raine A, Cheney RA, Ho R, et al. Nutritional supplementation to reduce child aggression: a randomized, stratified, single-blind, factorial trial. J Child Psychol Psychiatry. 2016;57(9):1038-1046.

7.      Hale MW, Spencer SJ, Conti B, et al. Diet, behavior and immunity across the lifespan. Neurosci Biobehav Rev. 2015;58:46-62.

Between the years 2010 and 2030, the population of the United States over 65 years of age will increase by 73%. One out of every five Americans will be over 65 at that time. Between 1900 and 2000, the total US population increased 3 times but the population of people 65 years or older increased more than 10 times. The growth rate for the population 65 years or older is expected to outpace that for the total population during the next several decades. By 2040, the percentage of elderly patients will increase 20%. Elderly patients in the United States are estimated to be 55 million by 2020 and 80 million by 2040.

Pain management in elderly patients can be a challenge. Elderly patients can be taking many different medications. Some of these drugs can adversely interact with some pain medications. Senile patients may forget to take their medications as prescribed. Their kidneys do not function as well as in younger patients.

Your kidneys are responsible for eliminating drugs. As a result, drugs like morphine can accumulate within an elderly patient's body which could cause an overdose. Your liver metabolizes (breaks down drugs). Some elderly patients cannot afford some medications and therefore do not take them.

Liver function can also be compromised in elderly patients. This decreased function can affect the breakdown of many drugs. An elderly patient's body mass may be decreased as well. As a result, there is less body volume where a drug can go. A dose of drug will be distributed through various body tissues. If you are emaciated, a dose of drug will remain in your blood stream instead of being distributed throughout your body. As a result, the concentration of drug in your blood stream may be higher than expected.

Your kidneys become smaller with age. As a result, there is decreased blood flow to the kidney and less effective filtration with removal of a drug from the kidney. As one ages, the liver undergoes a decrease in mass and blood flow. Decreased saliva noted in some older patients may interfere with swallowing. Drugs prescribed by mouth may be absorbed differently because of changes in stomach acid levels in older patients. The changes in physiology with aging may alter the side effect profile of many drugs.

One other important consideration is that of elderly persons being able to adequately monitor and adhere to their own scheduled pharmacological administration. Elderly patients may skip medication doses or cut them in half. Because pain is very common among the elderly, all elderly patients should be asked about their pain. Chronic pain can lead to depression, and polypharmacy. The cause of an elderly patient's pain may be difficult to identify and may be multifactorial. Inadequate treatment of pain is common among elderly patients. Thus, psychosocial support and nondrug treatments that reduce pain are particularly important. Patient and caregiver education and active caregiver involvement can help reduce pain and improve quality of life.

The prevalence of pain in elderly patients is higher among nursing home residents. In elderly patients, the most common sites of pain are joints, and the most common causes of pain are musculoskeletal disorders. Cancer related pain is not infrequent. Psychological factors such as depression and anxiety can prolong or amplify pain. The effect of age on pain perception is unknown. Perception may be influenced by many sociologic factors.

Chronic pain is characterized by a vague onset. The cause is often a chronic disorder. Sometimes the cause is clear, but the pain lasts longer than the expected time for healing. Neuropathic pain often manifests as spontaneous burning pain with superimposed lancinating pain. Neuropathic pain tends to follow the distribution of a neural pathway. Chronic pain in elderly patients may gradually lead to insomnia, decreased appetite, weight loss and constipation. Patients may become preoccupied with physical symptoms, become inactive, and withdraw socially.

Depression is common in older patients. Inactivity can lead to deconditioning. Many elderly patients take pain for granted and do not mention it unless they are asked. The assessment of patients with impaired cognition may be challenging.

Patients with dementia may be able to describe their current symptoms but unable to reliably report their previous symptoms. Depression, secondary gain, personality disorders, and psychological stress should be evaluated in all elderly patients.

The patient's physical examination should focus on the musculoskeletal system and include palpation for trigger points, evaluation for joint swelling and inflammation, and evaluation for pain with passive range of motion. Pain is suggested by facial grimacing, frowning, or repetitive eye blinking. In the elderly, pain often has multiple causes, and no single predominant cause can be identified.

Poor pain management decreases the patient's quality of life and may contribute to suicide. The elderly are more likely than younger patients to experience adverse effects of analgesics. Drug dosing starting low and going upward slowly. Oral analgesic administration is usually preferred because it is convenient and results in relatively steady blood levels.

Acetaminophen is the analgesic of choice for most elderly people with mild to moderate pain. Despite its relative lack of anti-inflammatory activity, acetaminophen is usually the best drug for initial treatment of osteoarthritis. NSAIDs are indicated when inflammation contributes significantly to pain. Adverse effects vary, and a patient may tolerate one NSAID better than another. NSAIDs tend to have a ceiling analgesic dose.

The most common adverse effect of all NSAIDs is gastrointestinal upset, which may require stopping the drug. Ulceration and GI bleeding can occur. Ulceration with or without bleeding can occur simultaneously or independently of each other. Risk of ulcers and GI bleeding for people 65 years or over is 3 to 4 times higher than that for middle-aged people.

NSAIDs can impair renal function and cause sodium and water retention; they should be used cautiously in the elderly, particularly in those who have a renal disorder. Nonacetylated salicylates may have less renal toxicity and fewer antiplatelet effects than other NSAIDs.

Opioids are the most potent analgesics. Opioids act by blocking receptors in the brain and spinal cord. In the elderly, opioids have an increased half-life and possibly a greater analgesic effect than in younger patients. Nonetheless, the most common error in prescribing these drugs is to give them too infrequently, allowing breakthrough pain.

A few opioids have specific advantages and disadvantages in elderly patients. Fentanyl causes less histamine release and thus less vasodilation and hypotension. Meperidine should be avoided in elderly patients. Meperidine is less effective when given orally and can cause confusion; also, it is metabolized to an active form that tends to accumulate and thus may lead to central nervous system excitement and seizures.

Opioid agonist-antagonists, which have both agonist and antagonist effects on opiate receptors, often have psychotomimetic effects in the elderly. For this reason, pentazocine (Talwin) and butorphanol (Stadol) are rarely appropriate for the elderly patient. The analgesic effect of propoxyphene (Darvon) which is no longer available is similar to that of aspirin or acetaminophen, but dependency and renal impairment may occur.

As a result, propoxyphene should not be used in the elderly. In patients with renal insufficiency, excretion of morphine and codeine may be delayed, resulting in undesirably long therapeutic or adverse effects, particularly with sustained-release formulations. In these patients, hydromorphone or oxycodone is less likely to accumulate and may be preferred.

Opioids can be given transdermally (on your skin). However, transdermal fentanyl should be used only in patients who have already been stabilized on opioids. Transdermal fentanyl is long-lasting. The peak analgesic effect of transdermal fentanyl occurs 18 to 24 h after application.

If this drug is used, a rapid-onset analgesic is required in the meantime. It is important to know that the reservoir for this system is the skin and not in the patch. If an overdose occurs, removing the patch does little to stop drug delivery within the first 18 h after removal.

Patients must be closely observed if they have a fever. A fever can cause an increased uptake of the drug into the elderly patient's body. As a result an overdose could occur.

A heating pad can also cause a fentanyl overdose. Continuous opioid infusion provides steady-state analgesic drug levels. This means that there are no peaks and valleys in the elderly patient's bloodstream. Continuous infusion in palliative care patients may also be useful if regional techniques and NSAIDs are ineffective or inappropriate in patients near the end of life.

Patient-controlled analgesia enables a patient to increase drug delivery as needed. This technique results in a more stable blood drug level, thus avoiding the roller-coaster effects of intramuscular dosing. Patient-controlled analgesia reduces overall drug use and has fewer adverse side effects. However, patients with confusion or dementia cannot effectively use patient-controlled analgesia.

Opioid muscle injection is rarely used. Initially, drug blood levels are high, resulting in more frequent adverse effects. The blood drug levels decrease rapidly, resulting in pain recurrence.

Unlike NSAIDS, opioids have no ceiling analgesic effect as dosage is increased. The maximum dose is whatever is needed to relieve pain. However, adverse effects may limit the maximum dose that is used. Opioids cause dose-related sedation and respiratory depression.

Most elderly patients taking opioids should not drive and should take precautions to prevent falls. Opioids may cause confusion. If confusion is due to an opioid, pupils are usually very constricted. Sometimes decreasing the dose may relieve confusion without significantly decreasing analgesia. If this approach is ineffective, a different analgesic may be necessary.

Opioids almost always cause constipation or urinary retention. Patients do not develop tolerance to these adverse effects. When an opioid is started, the patient's intake of fluid and fiber should be increased to try to prevent constipation. If a laxative is needed, a fiber laxative may be used.

Gabapentin (Neurontin) is frequently prescribed in elderly patients. Dose reductions of gabapentin are recommended in patients with renal insufficiency. Dizziness and drowsiness are common adverse effects. Pregabilin (Lyrica) is frequently in elderly patients with post herpetic neuralgia.

Antidepressant medications are also prescribed as adjunct medications for elderly patients who suffer from pain. For tricyclic antidepressants, amitriptyline, which is highly sedating and anticholinergic, should be avoided in the elderly. Local anesthetics injected into painful muscle areas are sometimes effective.

Local anesthetics injected into joints can relieve joint pain as well. Topical drugs are frequently used for pain originating in peripheral nerves. Capsaicin cream, NSAID creams, or a Lidoderm (lidocaine 5%) patch should be considered as well.

Physical therapy can reduce pain due to musculoskeletal disorders in elderly patients. Aquatic therapy can help muscle and joint pain. Pain due to muscle spasm may be reduced by stretching, muscle massages, cold therapy or heat therapy.

Ultrasound therapy may relieve musculoskeletal pain originating in your deep tissues. Transcutaneous electrical nerve stimulation (TENS) can relieve many types of pain as well. Alternative therapies are also used by many patients to control their pain. Occupational therapy can be helpful as well.

Given that no two people are alike, if you are taking any medications and begin to take nutritional supplements you should be aware that potential drug-nutrient interactions may occur and are encouraged to consult a health care professional before using any natural product. Combining certain prescription drugs and dietary supplements can lead to undesirable effects such as: diminished prescription drug effectiveness, reduced supplement effectiveness and impaired drug and/or supplement absorption.

Ginger powder supplementation at a dose of 1 g/d can reduce inflammatory markers in elderly patients with knee osteoarthritis, and it thus can be recommended as a suitable supplement for these patients.[1]

In elderly patients with a fracture of the distal radius, administration of the probiotic could greatly accelerating the healing process.[2] Soy protein (SP) may be of benefit in the management of osteoarthritis (OA) in men but not women. Examining and verifying the long-term effects of SP on improving symptoms of OA, particularly in men, is warranted.[3]

A study was done to evaluate whether vitamin D status modifies the association between statin use and musculoskeletal pain. These findings support the hypothesis that vitamin D deficiency modifies the risk of musculoskeletal symptoms experienced with statin use.4

References

1.      Naderi Z, Mozaffari-Khosravi H, Dehghan A, Nadjarzadeh A, Huseini HF. Effect of ginger powder supplementation on nitric oxide and C-reactive protein in elderly knee osteoarthritis patients: A 12-week double-blind randomized placebo-controlled clinical trial. J Tradit Complement Med. 2016;6(3):199-203.

2.      Lei M, Hua LM, Wang DW. The effect of probiotic treatment on elderly patients with distal radius fracture: a prospective double-blind, placebo-controlled randomised clinical trial. Benef Microbes. 2016:1-8.

3.      Arjmandi BH, Khalil DA, Lucas EA, et al. Soy protein may alleviate osteoarthritis symptoms. Phytomedicine. 2004;11(7-8):567-575.

4.      Morioka TY, Lee AJ, Bertisch S, Buettner C. Vitamin D status modifies the association between statin use and musculoskeletal pain: a population based study. Atherosclerosis. 2015;238(1):77-82.

Palliative Care is a relatively new medical specialty. The goal of palliative care is to improve the quality of life for patients as well as their families. Palliative care is appropriate at any point in an illness. Palliative care can be provided at the same time as conventional treatment that is meant to cure you. Palliative care is dedicated to maximizing a person's comfort, independence, and quality of life when the prolongation of life is no longer a realistic goal. More than 50% of dying patients do not receive adequate symptomatic relief. Fear of hastening death is the primary reason for physicians' reluctance to prescribe high-dose pain medication.

Palliative care is the active total care of patients whose disease is not amenable to curative treatment. Control of a patient's pain and other symptoms, and of psychological, social, and spiritual problems is mandatory. The goal is achievement of the best possible quality of life for patients and their families.

Palliative care aims to relieve symptoms such as pain, shortness of breath, fatigue, constipation, nausea, loss of appetite and difficulty sleeping. It helps patients gain the strength to carry on with daily life. It improves their ability to tolerate medical treatments. And it helps them better understand their choices for care. The goal of palliative care is to offer patients the best possible quality of life during their illness.

Palliative care is not the same as hospice care. Palliative care may be provided at any time during a person's illness, even from the time of diagnosis. And, it may be given at the same time as curative treatment. Hospice care always includes palliative care. However, it is focused on terminally ill patients-people who no longer seek treatments to cure them and who are expected to live for about six months or less. Palliative care affirms life and regards dying as a normal natural process. It neither hastens nor postpones death.

Palliative care provides relief from pain and psychological symptoms. Its goal is to integrate the psychological and spiritual aspects of a patient's care. It offers a support system to help patients live as actively as possible until their death. It offers a support system to help families cope during the patient's illness.

Palliative care is not provided by one physician but by a team of experts, including palliative care doctors, nurses and social workers. Chaplains, neuropaths, massage therapists, pharmacists, nutritionists and others are also a part of the team. Palliative care can be provided when you are at home, in an assisted living facility, nursing facility or hospital. Palliative care in contrast to hospice care is not just for patients who are very close to death.

Palliative care is therefore, more than health care just for dying persons. Palliative care is a health care philosophy aimed at improving the essence of life when cure is no longer possible. Palliative care is a health care discipline with its own research knowledge base and a specific set of skills aimed at pain and other forms of suffering which becomes the major focus of treatment.

The American Board of Anesthesiology has subspecialty certification in palliative care. Palliative care is totally defined by prognosis but by what it inspires, offers, and achieves. A patient does not have to be dying to have palliative care. Palliative care is in addition to providing medical care, is also a provider of paramedical support services. Palliative care ensures informed choices be offered to patients.

The management of pain is an important aspect of palliative care. The patient must be regarded as a living person and therefore the full human experiences; physical, emotional, and spiritual, must be addressed. A patient must not die with severe pain. The patient must be comfortable.

Most important a patient must be able to live out his or hers last moment as fully and consciously as possible. In fact palliative care should make dying to be a patient's finest hour. A dying patient is unique and should be treated as someone special.

Palliative care is any form of medical care or treatment that concentrates on reducing the severity of disease symptoms rather than trying to seek a cure. The goal is to prevent and relieve suffering and to improve quality of life for people facing serious, complex illnesses. It should not be confused with hospice care which delivers palliative care to those at the end of life. In essence, palliative care provides care to those with life limiting illness at any stage of their disease.

Given that no two people are alike, if you are taking any medications and begin to take nutritional supplements you should be aware that potential drug-nutrient interactions may occur and are encouraged to consult a health care professional before using any natural product. Combining certain prescription drugs and dietary supplements can lead to undesirable effects such as: diminished prescription drug effectiveness, reduced supplement effectiveness and impaired drug and/or supplement absorption.

The foundations of good nutrition, exercise, stress reduction, and reengagement in life can contribute much to restoring the quality of life to a pain patient.[1]

Nutrition in palliative care and at the end of life should be one of the goals for improving quality of life.[2] It is important to address issues of food and feeding at this time to assist in the management of troublesome symptoms as well as to enhance the remaining life. Cancer and its treatments exert a major impact upon physical and psychological reserves and at the end of life problems with appetite and the ability to eat and drink compound such impact.

Previous studies have shown that the dietary habits of cancer patients and survivors have significant implications for their recovery and quality of life.[3] Nutrition and eating behaviors have a significant effect on cancer patients' physical and emotional adjustment.

The aims of nutritional care minimize food-related discomfort and maximize food enjoyment. Ethical questions will be raised concerning the provision of food and fluids to a person nearing the end of their life. Nurses need to acknowledge that food has greater significance than the provision of nutrients.

References

1.      Dillard JN, Knapp S. Complementary and alternative pain therapy in the emergency department. Emerg Med Clin North Am. 2005;23(2):529-549.

2.      Acreman S. Nutrition in palliative care. Br J Community Nurs. 2009;14(10):427-428, 430-421.

3.      Barak-Nahum A, Haim LB, Ginzburg K. When life gives you lemons: The effectiveness of culinary group intervention among cancer patients. Soc Sci Med. 2016;166:1-8.

A high level of malnutrition has been reported in adults in hospital and is linked to poor clinical outcome. Almost 50% of patients are malnourished on hospital admission. Many others develop malnutrition during admission. Malnutrition contributes to hospital morbidity, mortality, costs, and readmissions.

Malnutrition is an under-recognized problem in hospitalized patients. Nutrition support is recognized as an important cofactor in altering morbidity and mortality of hospitalized patients. Malnutrition in hospitals remains a serious issue. It occurs worldwide and affects patients of all ages. Almost 50% of patients are malnourished on hospital admission; many others develop malnutrition during admission.

The prevalence of malnutrition for older adults (>65 years) in hospital and rehabilitation units has been reported as being as high as 60%; some older patients with good appetites do not receive sufficient nourishment because of inadequate feeding assistance.

Malnutrition contributes to hospital morbidity, mortality, costs, and readmissions. The Joint Commission requires malnutrition risk screening on admission. Disease states and acute events predispose patients to malnutrition, the degree of which is usually determined by the severity of the illness.

The Joint Commission requires malnutrition risk screening on admission. If screening identifies malnutrition risk, a nutrition assessment is required to create a nutrition care plan. The Joint Commission has mandated universal screening and assessment of hospitalized patients for malnutrition since 1995.

The plan should be initiated early in the hospital course, as even patients with normal nutrition become malnourished quickly when acutely ill. Patients with inadequate intake over time may develop potentially fatal refeeding syndrome.

The hospitalist must be able to recognize the risk factors for malnutrition, patients at risk of refeeding syndrome, and the optimal route for nutrition support. Finally, education of patients and their caregivers about nutrition support must begin before discharge, and include coordination of care with outpatient facilities.[1]

Malnutrition in hospitals remains a serious issue. It occurs worldwide and affects patients of all ages. Patients who are at risk for malnutrition-related complications (MRCs) must be identified.[2] The characteristics that correlated best with malnutrition-related complications risk level assignment were occurrence of a wound, poor oral intake, malnutrition-related admission diagnosis, serum albumin value, hemoglobin value, and total lymphocyte count.

A model using four variables (malnutrition-related admission diagnosis, serum albumin value, hemoglobin value, and total lymphocyte count) was almost as good as that using six predictors. The ability of admission information to accurately reflect MRC risk is crucial to early initiation of restorative medical nutritional therapy.

For years, physicians have attempted to improve the metabolic status of patients after surgery or trauma. Currently, major emphasis is placed on perioperative nutritional status and its effect on postoperative wound healing.

It is suggested that the issue of nutrition in hospitals is of concern and that there are numerous factors which contribute to this. However, this aspect of patient care is not identified as the specific responsibility of hospital staff. Nurses should play a pivotal role in preventing malnutrition in hospital but, in most cases, they do not.[3]

Vague musculoskeletal complaints in these chronically ill patients may be attributed to multiple underlying disease processes rather than a deficiency in vitamin D.[4] some hospital formularies continue to provide multivitamin supplements that contain less vitamin D than currently is recommended.

Hypovitaminosis C and D are highly prevalent in acutely hospitalized patients, but the clinical significance of these biochemical abnormalities is not known. Because deficiencies of vitamin C and D have been linked to psychologic abnormalities, vitamin C or D provision could improve the mood state of acutely hospitalized patients. Treatment of hypovitaminosis C improves the mood state of acutely hospitalized patients.[5]

Unintentional weight loss is used as a reliable indicator of malnutrition. Peripheral parenteral nutrition is an alternative when caloric intake is impossible or insufficient or refused by the patient, as it minimizes the complications of the central catheter.

Serum phosphate levels are associated with anemia in hospitalized patients. Maintaining optimal phosphate reduces the likelihood of anemia and whether ideal phosophate during acute care hospitalization influences clinical outcomes.[6]

Nutritional support should be considered in people who are malnourished, as defined by any of the following: A body mass index (BMI) of less than 18.5 kg/m2, unintentional weight loss greater than 10% within the preceding 3-6 months, and A BMI of less than 20 kg/m$^2$ .

The most obvious medical conditions that contribute to malnutrition include those that are those that prevent oral food intake, such as oral cancer, tumors or strictures in the throat or esophagus, stroke, and degenerative neurologic disorders that result in dysphagia.

Trauma patients and others who are ventilator dependent rely on the timely initiation of nutrition support. Conditions such as chronic obstructive pulmonary disease, chronic infections, and cancer can result in increased metabolic demand and weight loss due to cachexia and poor oral intake.

Any patient identified to be at risk should have a nutrition assessment, using information on weight and weight changes, food intake, gastrointestinal symptoms, functional capacity, disease state, physical characteristics, and symptoms of micronutrient deficiencies. There is increasing awareness that chronic wound healing is very dependent on the patient's nutritional status.

The anesthesiologist's involvement in perioperative medicine has significantly changed. In order to identify patients at risks of perioperative complications, the anesthesiologist has to consider, amongst others, screening and management of undernutrition. In other words, the anesthesiologist could play an important role in undernutrition screening and its management in order to reduce perioperative morbidity.

With the move to a more integrated curriculum and problem-based learning at many medical schools, a substantial portion of the total nutrition instruction is occurring outside courses specifically dedicated to nutrition. The amount of nutrition education in medical schools remains inadequate.[7]

The primary mission of the Nutrition in Medicine (NIM) project is to provide tools to facilitate the nutrition training of undergraduate medical students. These innovative strategies should allow a better fit of NIM within diverse medical school environments and help to promote incorporation of the curriculum into more medical schools.[8]

References

1.     Kirkland LL, Kashiwagi DT, Brantley S, Scheurer D, Varkey P. Nutrition in the hospitalized patient. J Hosp Med. 2013;8(1):52-58.

2.     Brugler L, Stankovic AK, Schlefer M, Bernstein L. A simplified nutrition screen for hospitalized patients using readily available laboratory and patient information. Nutrition. 2005;21(6):650-658.

3.     Cortis JD. Nutrition and the hospitalized patient: implications for nurses. Br J Nurs. 1997;6(12):666-667, 670-664.

4.        Lyman D. Undiagnosed vitamin D deficiency in the hospital-ized patient. Am Fam Physician. 2005;71(2):299-304.

5.        Zhang M, Robitaille L, Eintracht S, Hoffer LJ. Vitamin C provision improves mood in acutely hospitalized patients. Nutrition. 2011;27(5):530-533.

6.        Otero TM, Canales C, Yeh DD, et al. Association of Serum Phosphate Levels and Anemia in Critically Ill Surgical Patients. JPEN J Parenter Enteral Nutr. 2016.

7.        Adams KM, Lindell KC, Kohlmeier M, Zeisel SH. Status of nutrition education in medical schools. Am J Clin Nutr. 2006;83(4):941S-944S.

8.        Lindell KC, Adams KM, Kohlmeier M, Zeisel SH. The evo-lution of Nutrition in Medicine, a computer-assisted nutrition curriculum. Am J Clin Nutr. 2006;83(4):956S-962S.

Food provides information to the body, signaling basic biological functions and normalizing physiological processes. Despite the complexity of the correlation between diet and disease, there is now a sufficient body of evidence to encourage applying nutritional science in everyday clinical practice. The foods you eat render your chronic pain worse, or better.

The fundamental principle nutrition is that patients with chronic pain need a high protein intake diet with avoidance of sugars and starches. High cholesterol, lipids, and glucose are almost universal in patients with uncontrolled pain.

Agricultural biotechnology and genetically modified (GM) crops are effective tools to substantially increase productivity, quality, and environmental sustainability in agricultural farming. Furthermore, they may contribute to improving the nutritional content of crops, addressing needs related to public health.[1]

There is not sufficient evidence in medical literature to support claims that organic food is safer or healthier than conventionally grown food. Properly used in this agricultural science context, "organic" refers to the methods grown and processed, not necessarily the chemical composition of the food. Foods claiming to be organic must be free of artificial food additives, and are often processed with fewer artificial methods, materials and conditions, such as chemical ripening, food irradiation, and genetically modified ingredients.

The Environmental Protection Agency maintains strict guidelines on the regulation of pesticides by setting a tolerance on the amount of pesticide residue allowed to be in or on any particular food. The main difference between organic and conventional food products are the chemicals involved during production and processing

Organic meat certification in the United States requires farm animals to be raised according to USDA organic regulations throughout their lives. These regulations require that livestock are fed certified organic food that contains no animal byproducts. Further, organic farm animals can receive no growth hormones or antibiotics, and they must be raised using techniques that protect native species and other natural resources. Irradiation and genetic engineering are not allowed with organic animal production.

Genetically modified foods or GM foods, also genetically engineered foods, are foods produced from organisms that have had changes introduced into their DNA using the methods of genetic engineering. Genetically modified crops have been engineered for resistance to pathogens and herbicides and for better nutrient profiles. Genetically modified livestock are organisms from the group of cattle, sheep, pigs, goats, birds, horses and fish kept for human consumption, whose genetic material (DNA) has been altered using genetic engineering techniques.

Chronically low levels of nutrients or imbalances among nutrients can inhibit essential biochemical reactions and plant the seeds for degenerative diseases later in life. Kale, spinach, dark green lettuces and other greens contain extensive amounts of alpha-linolenic acid, which is the building block of the omega-3 fatty acids.

Protein contains the amino acids that are critical for many pain control functions, including formation of many neurotransmitters, hormones, muscle, and cartilage. Dietary counseling must be a component of chronic pain care. The scientific literature contains plenty of data indicating a strong link between chronic pain and nutrition

Gluten, found in all products made from wheat, rye, barley, spelt and hidden in many other products, such as soy sauce, corn muffins, etc., causes inflammation in the body. The vast majority of dietary carbohydrates and calories come from highly refined grains such as wheat, corn and rye, and sugars (sucrose and high-fructose corn syrup, in soft drinks and other beverages, and fried potatoes.

Sugar is highly inflammatory and is found in almost all processed foods. Replace all processed food with whole food. If a food has a list of ingredients, you should not eat it. Instead eat vegetables, fruits, nuts, and organic, free range animal protein. Alcohol, cigarettes, sugar products and soft drinks may all cause inflammation which increases your pain. Pastry, bread cookies, etc. may contribute to obesity. Obesity contributes to inflammation as well. Pain is caused by injury, infection, irritation, ischemia and inflammation. Injury, irritation, ischemia and infection cause inflammation. Inflammation is the body's way of healing the body. However when inflammation becomes chronic, it causes chronic pain which is difficult to control.

No single food can completely stop chronic pain, but a healthful diet is a powerful part of your pain-management strategy. The Mediterranean diet, for example, is rich in fruits and vegetables, whole grains, and healthful unsaturated fats. Eat salmon, mackerel, herring, sardines as well as sea algae. Fish provides the proper balance of Essential Fatty Acids which naturally lubricate joints and muscles and reduce inflammation.

Eat oils such from nuts, avocados, olives, olive oil, hemp and flax seed oil. These oils lubricate also lubricate joints and muscles and reduce inflammation. Turmeric, black pepper and ginger are known for reducing inflammation and pain.

Many individuals are allergic to gluten, causing what is known as celiac disease. In these people, eating gluten triggers an inflammatory response, which primarily attacks tacks the gastrointestinal tract and interferes with vitamin and mineral absorption. Gluten sensitivity may appear as immunological reactions affecting the nervous system, balance, and behavior, as well as a person's overall sense of well-being. Lectins play a role in rheumatoid arthritis and possibly other inflammatory autoimmune diseases.

Chronically low levels of nutrients or imbalances among nutrients can inhibit essential biochemical reactions and plant the seeds for degenerative diseases later in life. Kale, spinach, dark green lettuces and other greens contain extensive amounts of alpha-linolenic acid, which is the building block of the omega-3 fatty acids.

Foods that may help control chronic pain in conditions such as fibromyalgia and rheumatoid arthritis include cherries, soy, oranges, peaches, asparagus, cranberries, cauliflower and kiwi. In the case of an inflammatory illness such as rheumatoid arthritis, dairy products, chocolate, eggs, meat, wheat, corn and nuts can theoretically worsen inflammation.

Eating foods that contain saturated fats raises the level of cholesterol in your blood. High levels of LDL cholesterol in your blood increase your risk of heart disease and stroke. From a chemical standpoint, saturated fats are simply fat molecules that have no double bonds between carbon molecules because they are saturated with hydrogen molecules. Saturated fats are typically solid at room temperature. Replacing foods that are high in saturated fat with healthier options can lower blood cholesterol levels and improve lipid profiles.

Eicosanoids are a group of biochemicals in your body that signal oxidation. Arachidonic acid is an example. These chemicals cause chronic pain. Prostaglandins, thromboxane leukotrienes etc.are also examples of eiconosoids. They cause pain, inflammation, allergy, hypertension, etc. Proper nutrition may decrease some of these effects.

Saturated fats occur naturally in many foods. The majority come mainly from animal sources, including meat and dairy products. Examples are: fatty beef, lamb, pork, poultry with skin, beef fat (tallow),lard and cream, butter, cheese and other dairy products made from whole or reduced-fat (2 percent) milk. In addition, many baked goods and fried foods can contain high levels of saturated fats. Some plant-based oils, such as palm oil, palm kernel oil and coconut oil, also contain primarily saturated fats, but do not contain cholesterol.

To get the nutrients you need, eat a dietary pattern that emphasizes: fruits, vegetables, whole grains, low-fat dairy products, poultry, fish and nuts, while limiting red meat and sugary foods and beverages. You should replace foods high in saturated fats with foods high in monounsaturated and/or polyunsaturated fats. This means eating foods made with liquid vegetable oil but not tropical oils. It also means eating fish and nuts. You also might try to replace some of the meat you eat with beans or legumes. The American Heart Association recommends limiting saturated fats which are found in butter, cheese, red meat and other animal based foods.

There are two main types of potentially harmful dietary fat: trans-fat and saturated fat. Saturated fat is a type of fat that comes mainly from animal sources of food, such as red meat, poultry and full-fat dairy products. Saturated fat raises total blood cholesterol levels and low-density lipoprotein (LDL) cholesterol levels, which can increase your risk of cardiovascular disease. Saturated fat may also increase your risk of type 2 diabetes.

When chickens are housed indoors and deprived of greens, their meat and eggs also become artificially low in omega-3s. Eggs from pastured hens can contain as much as 10 times more omega-3s than eggs from factory hens.

Trans fat is a type of fat that occurs naturally in some foods in small amounts. But most trans fats are made from oils through a food processing method called partial hydrogenation. These partially hydrogenated trans fats can increase unhealthy LDL cholesterol and lower healthy high-density lipoprotein (HDL) cholesterol. This can increase your risk of cardiovascular disease.

Most fats that have a high percentage of saturated fat or that contain trans-fat are solid at room temperature. Because of this, they're typically referred to as solid fats. They include beef fat, pork fat, butter, shortening and stick margarine. The types of potentially helpful dietary fat are mostly unsaturated.

Monounsaturated fatty acids are a type of fat found in a variety of foods and oils. Studies show that eating foods rich in monounsaturated fatty acids improves blood cholesterol levels, which can decrease your risk of heart disease. Research also shows that these fatty acids may benefit insulin levels and blood sugar control, which can be especially helpful if you have type 2 diabetes.

Polyunsaturated fatty acids are a type of fat found mostly in plant-based foods and oils. Evidence shows that eating foods rich in polyunsaturated fatty acids improves blood cholesterol levels, which can decrease your risk of heart disease. These fatty acids may also help decrease the risk of type 2 diabetes.

Omega-3 fatty acids are one type of polyunsaturated fat is made up of mainly omega-3 fatty acids and may be especially beneficial to your heart. Omega-3, found in some types of fatty fish, appears to decrease the risk of coronary artery disease. There are plant sources of omega-3 fatty acids. However, it hasn't yet been determined whether replacements for fish oil plant-based or krill have the same health effects as omega-3 fatty acid from fish.

Foods made up mostly of monounsaturated and polyunsaturated fats are liquid at room temperature, such as olive oil, safflower oil, peanut oil and corn oil. Fish are high in omega-3 fatty acids and include salmon, tuna, trout, mackerel, sardines and herring. Plant sources of omega-3 fatty acids include flaxseed, oils (canola, flaxseed, soybean), and nuts and other seeds (walnuts, butternuts and sunflower). It's more important to eat beneficial  fats and avoid harmful fats. Fat is an important part of a healthy diet. Avoid trans fat.

Unsaturated fats lower disease risk. Trans fats increase disease risk, even when eaten in small quantities. Foods containing trans fats are primarily in processed foods made with trans-fat from partially hydrogenated oil. Saturated fats, while not as harmful as trans fats, by comparison with unsaturated fats negatively impact health and are best consumed in moderation.

A free-range chicken is a bird that is allowed constant access to the outdoors, with plenty of fresh vegetation, sunshine and room to exercise. Moreover, it has not been given any chemicals (antibiotics, for example) of any kind. According to the USDA's official standards, 'free-range' means little more than chickens having occasional access to the outside world.

What some producers and farmers call "pastured" chicken is much more in line what with many people think they're getting with free range. They might be fed grain as well, but they have access to a greater variety of food in their diet, and the result is much more richly flavored meat and eggs. It's also much more expensive to raise chickens this way, because of the amount of space required and how that limits how many chickens you might be able to raise at a time.

Natural chicken means that nothing has been added to the bird after slaughter. This means that no flavoring, brines, coloring, etc. has been added. The USDA requires marketers to say specifically what they mean when they use the term, such as "no artificial flavors".

Certified organic, means that the animal been grown in a field that has not seen chemical fertilizers, fungicides, herbicides or genetically modified organisms for at least three years. Antibiotics are not allowed at all.

With the increased global production of different genetically modified (GM) plant varieties, chances increase that unauthorized GM organisms (UGMOs) may enter the food chain. At the same time, the detection of UGMOs is a challenging task because of the limited sequence information that will generally be available.[2]

Genetically modified food is able to oppose the world's hunger and preserve the environment, even if the patents in this matter are symptomatic of several doubts. And also, transgenic consumption causes problems and skepticism among consumers in several European countries, but above all in Italy, where there is a strong opposition over recent years.[3]

Long-term feeding corn carrying cry1Ac genes to Wuzhishan miniature pigs did not indicate adverse effects on the growth, immune response and health indicators at any stages of growth.[4] The ability to manipulate and customize the genetic code of living organisms has brought forth the production of genetically modified organisms (GMOs) and consumption of genetically modified (GM) foods.[5]

Studies on the long-term health effects of GM plants, including tests of mutagenicity, teratogenicity and carcinogenicity seem to be still clearly necessary.[6] Genetically modified soya bean (GMSB) is a commercialized food. It has been shown to have adverse effects on fertility in animal trials.[7] Current research has shown that GM foods do not cause increased allergenicity or have a meaningful risk of gene transfer to people.[8]

Grass-fed beef and dairy products are leaner, but more importantly, lower in omega-6 fats that are linked to heart disease. Grass-fed meat and dairy products also are higher in beneficial omega-3 fats and conjugated linoleic acids. Both reduce the risk of heart disease. Meat from grass-fed animals has two to four times more omega-3 fatty acids than meat from grain-fed animals.

Clinical experience suggests that fasting followed by vegetarian diet may help patients with rheumatoid arthritis (RA). Available evidence suggests that fasting followed by vegetarian diets might be useful in the treatment of RA.[9] Some patients with RA can benefit from a fasting period followed by a vegetarian diet. Thus, dietary treatment may be a valuable adjunct to the ordinary therapeutic armamentarium for RA.[10]

It is suggested that a role for food allergy exists in at least some patients with rheumatic disease. A reduced ability to generate cytotaxins, reduced release of enzyme, and reduced leukotriene formation from RA neutrophils, together with an altered fatty acid composition of membrane phospholipids, may be mechanisms for the decrease of inflammatory symptoms that results from fasting.[11]

Dietary soy suppresses neuropathic pain in rats after partial sciatic nerve ligation. Some of the pain-suppression properties of soy can be attributed to phytoestrogens, isoflavones abundantly found in soy products. Average, but not low or high, plasma levels of phytoestrogens are associated with analgesia.

Overproduction of proinflammatory cytokines is a main trait of rheumatoid arthritis. Coenzyme Q10 (CoQ10), an endogenous antioxidant, has shown anti-inflammatory effects in some diseases.[12] A study was performed to determine the effects of probiotic supplementation on clinical and metabolic status of patients with rheumatoid arthritis (RA).

The results of this study indicated that taking probiotic supplements for 8 weeks among patients with rheumatoid arthritis had beneficial effects on insulin levels, hs-CRP levels.[13]

Obesity, deficient nutrient intake, and poor eating behavior were highly prevalent in patients with chronic pain who underwent long-term opioid therapy[14] Chronic idiopathic pain syndromes are major causes of personal suffering, disability, and societal expense. Dietary n-6 linoleic acid has increased markedly in modern industrialized populations over the past century.

These high amounts of linoleic acid could hypothetically predispose to physical pain by increasing the production of pro-nociceptive linoleic acid-derived lipid autacoids and by interfering with the production of anti-nociceptive lipid autacoids derived from n-3 fatty acids.[15]

There appears to be a decentralization super sensitivity, as it is extended to different monoamines (5-HT, dopamine, noradrenaline, tyramine). This type of super sensitivity is compatible with the theory of a deficiency of neurotransmitters at the level of the anti-nociceptive and integrated systems, with subsequent central and peripheral super sensitivity.

A similar condition limited to the rostral section of the anti-nociceptive system is valid for the mechanism of idiopathic headache including migraine: central and peripheral super sensitivity to monoamines and opiates is also episodically observed in headache sufferers.[16]

Targeted analgesic dietary interventions are a promising strategy for alleviating pain and improving quality of life in patients with persistent pain syndromes, such as chronic daily headache (CDH). High intakes of the omega-6 (n-6) polyunsaturated fatty acids (PUFAs), linoleic acid (LA) and arachidonic acid (AA) may promote physical pain by increasing the abundance, and subsequent metabolism, of LA and AA in immune and nervous system tissues.[17] A dietary intervention increasing n-3 and reducing n-6 fatty acids reduced headache pain, altered antinociceptive lipid mediators, and improved quality-of-life in this patient population.

There is growing evidence that inflammation is an important mediator of pathophysiology in bipolar disorder. The omega-3 (n-3) and omega-6 (n-6) polyunsaturated fatty acid (PUFA) metabolic pathways participate in several inflammatory processes and have been linked through epidemiologic and clinical studies to bipolar disorder and its response to treatment.[18]

It is advisable to substitute polyunsaturated fats for saturated fats are a key component of worldwide dietary guidelines for coronary heart disease risk reduction and chest pain. There is worldwide dietary advice to substitute omega 6 linoleic acid or polyunsaturated fats in general, for saturated fats.[19]

References

1.      Sanchez MA, Leon G. Status of market, regulation and research of genetically modified crops in Chile. N Biotechnol. 2016;33(6):815-823.

2.      Arulandhu AJ, van Dijk JP, Dobnik D, et al. DNA enrichment approaches to identify unauthorized genetically modified organisms (GMOs). Anal Bioanal Chem. 2016;408(17):4575-4593.

3.      Boccia F, Sarnacchiaro P. Genetically Modified Foods and Consumer Perspective. Recent Pat Food Nutr Agric. 2015;7(1):28-34.

4.      Chen L, Sun Z, Liu Q, et al. Long-term toxicity study on genetically modified corn with cry1Ac gene in a Wuzhishan miniature pig model. J Sci Food Agric. 2016;96(12):4207-4214.

5.      Dizon F, Costa S, Rock C, Harris A, Husk C, Mei J. Genetically Modified (GM) Foods and Ethical Eating. J Food Sci. 2016;81(2):R287-291.

6.      Domingo JL. Safety assessment of GM plants: An updated review of the scientific literature. Food Chem Toxicol. 2016;95:12-18.

7.      El-Kholy TA, Al-Abbadi HA, Qahwaji D, et al. Ameliorating effect of olive oil on fertility of male rats fed on genetically modified soya bean. Food Nutr Res. 2015;59:27758.

8.      Finkelstein PE. Genetically Modified Foods: A Brief Overview of the Risk Assessment Process. GM Crops Food. 2016:0.

9.      Muller H, de Toledo FW, Resch KL. Fasting followed by vegetarian diet in patients with rheumatoid arthritis: a systematic review. Scand J Rheumatol. 2001;30(1):1-10.

10.     Kjeldsen-Kragh J. Rheumatoid arthritis treated with vegetarian diets. Am J Clin Nutr. 1999;70(3 Suppl):594S-600S.

11.    Hafstrom I, Ringertz B, Gyllenhammar H, Palmblad J, Harms-Ringdahl M. Effects of fasting on disease activity, neutrophil function, fatty acid composition, and leukotriene biosynthesis in patients with rheumatoid arthritis. Arthritis Rheum. 1988;31(5):585-592.

12.    Abdollahzad H, Aghdashi MA, Asghari Jafarabadi M, Alipour B. Effects of Coenzyme Q10 Supplementation on Inflammatory Cytokines (TNF-alpha, IL-6) and Oxidative Stress in Rheumatoid Arthritis Patients: A Randomized Controlled Trial. Arch Med Res. 2015;46(7):527-533.

13.    Zamani B, Golkar HR, Farshbaf S, et al. Clinical and metabolic response to probiotic supplementation in patients with rheumatoid arthritis: a randomized, double-blind, placebo-controlled trial. Int J Rheum Dis. 2016;19(9):869-879.

14.    Meleger AL, Froude CK, Walker J, 3rd. Nutrition and eating behavior in patients with chronic pain receiving long-term opioid therapy. PM R. 2014;6(1):7-12 e11.

15.    Ramsden CE, Ringel A, Majchrzak-Hong SF, et al. Dietary linoleic acid-induced alterations in pro- and anti-nociceptive lipid autacoids: Implications for idiopathic pain syndromes? Mol Pain. 2016;12.

16.    Sicuteri F, Fanciullacci M, Michelacci S. Decentralization supersensitivity in headache and central panalgesia. Res Clin Stud Headache. 1978;6:19-33.

17.    Ramsden CE, Mann JD, Faurot KR, et al. Low omega-6 vs. low omega-6 plus high omega-3 dietary intervention for chronic daily headache: protocol for a randomized clinical trial. Trials. 2011;12:97.

18.    Saunders EF, Ramsden CE, Sherazy MS, Gelenberg AJ, Davis JM, Rapoport SI. Omega-3 and Omega-6 Polyunsaturated Fatty Acids in Bipolar Disorder: A Review of Biomarker and Treatment Studies. J Clin Psychiatry. 2016;77(10):e1301-e1308.

19.    Ramsden CE, Zamora D, Leelarthaepin B, et al. Use of dietary linoleic acid for secondary prevention of coronary heart disease and death: evaluation of recovered data from the Sydney Diet Heart Study and updated meta-analysis. BMJ. 2013;346:e8707.

# Index

A neuropathy 167, 217

Acute pain 53

addiction 41, 43, 44, 45, 49, 50, 51, 52,
    53, 54

A-delta fibers. 7

anti-inflammatory drugs 15, 53, 59, 62,
    76, 123, 160, 162, 163, 164, 184, 185,
    194, 208, 236

arginine 72, 73, 197, 257, 258

axon 7

Benzodiazepines 69

bone scan 29, 37, 140, 176, 182, 201, 202,
    223, 228

buprenorphine 43

C fibers 7

Carpal tunnel syndrome 168

celiac disease 5, 281

Certified organic, 283

chronic daily headache 285

clonidine patch 94, 203

Cluster headaches 164

conversion disorder 260

C-reactive protein 3, 4, 30, 165, 270

Crohn's disease 106, 251, 252

denrite 7

diabetic neuropathy 76, 77, 78, 82, 169,
    173

Eicosanoids 23

EMG 29

EMLA 90, 91

erythrocyte sedimentation rate 30, 35

factitious disorders 261

fentanyl patch 44, 92, 93, 230

Gabapentin 76, 77, 78, 204, 268

Gate Control Theory 10

genetically modified 279, 283, 284, 286

Genetically modified food 284

Ginger powder 269

gluten 5, 154, 155, 281

highly refined grains 5

Hydromorphone 44, 45

Hypochondriasis 260

inflammation 1, 3, 4, 5, 7, 8, 13, 15, 23,
   25, 30, 35, 59, 60, 62, 64, 71, 80, 89,
   94, 95, 104, 123, 157, 163, 181, 183,
   184, 185, 196, 200, 204, 210, 213, 234,
   235, 237, 251, 252, 253, 256, 257, 258,
   266, 267, 280, 281, 285, 293

interleukin-6 4

irritable bowel syndrome 151, 249, 257,
   258

Ketamine 92

levorphanol 45

Lidoderm transdermal drug-delivery
   system 93

linoleic acid 3, 4, 165, 285, 286, 287

McGill pain questionnaire 27

Mediterranean Diet 238

metabolic syndrome 63, 73

Methadone 46, 49, 229

MRI 29

mucositis 257

Muscle relaxants 15, 66, 67, 68

myelogram 36

Narcotic drugs 41

Nerve Conduction Velocity tests 38

neuron 7

neuropathic pain 75, 76, 77, 79, 80, 171,
   218, 229, 284

Niacin 64, 171

ointments 87

omega-3 fatty acids 79, 84, 105, 165, 280,
   281, 282, 283, 284

omega-6 fatty acids 4, 13, 164, 262

Onion juice 178

Opioids 21, 41, 42, 43, 45, 50, 52, 267,
   268

oxymorphone 44, 230, 231

Pain is an unpleasant sensory and
  emotional experience following tissue
  injury. 1

Palliative care 271

polyphenol 56, 95, 187, 258

postherpetic neuralgia 76, 77, 197

pregabilin 76, 77, 194

Processed foods 4

Raynaud's disease 168, 233, 234, 236, 237

Resveratrol 95, 105

Saturated fat 84, 282

serotonin reuptake inhibitor 83

somatization disorder 259

Systemic lupus erythematosus 237

Tapentadol 46

TENS unit 16

Tietze's syndrome 246

Toradol 61

Tramadol 45

visceral pain 249

# About the Author

Dr. William E. Ackerman MD conveys considerable pain management experience. He is a clinician, academician, lecturer, author and researcher. Dr. Ackerman is: Board certified in Pain Medicine and Anesthesiology, is a Graduate of the University Of Louisville School Of Medicine, did a Residency in Anesthesiology at the University of Kentucky, and was Chief Resident in anesthesiology and Critical Care Medicine and did a Fellowship in Pain Medicine at the Texas Tech Health Sciences Center.

Dr. Ackerman was: nominated previously for the Southern Medical Society Medical Research Award, Bristol-Meyers Squibb award for distinguished achievement in Pain Research was a recipient of the Karl Koehler research grant from the American Society of Regional Anesthesia and Pain Medicine. He has been a Guest speaker at Medical school department meetings and academic symposiums throughout the country and at international meetings.

He published fifteen books and many chapters in multiple textbooks including the AMA best seller: The AMA Guides to Injury and Disease Causation (First and Second editions). He authored 135 scientific articles in prestigious medical journals such as: Anesthesia Analgesia, Canadian Journal of Anaesthesia, Regional Anesthesia and Pain Management, The Journal of Hand Surgery etc.

He was a Lt. Col in the US Army and Chief of Anesthesiology of two Army medical Center Hospitals and was director of pain management at two private hospitals. Dr. Ackerman was Director of Pain Management at a University Hospital pain clinic and was an Associate Professor. He was director of pain management at two private hospitals and was selected to "Who's Who in International Medicine".

Dr. Ackerman has expertise in the treatment of a variety of painful conditions including neck, back, neuropathic, shingles, joint pain, fibromyalgia, myofascial pain, RSD, whiplash and cancer pain.

He emphasizes proper nutrition, smoking cessation as well as exercise in addition to the standard pain management modalities. A poor diet, cigarette smoking and obesity contribute to chronic inflammation which in turn contributes to chronic pain. These are the factors which prompted him to write this book.

www.ingramcontent.com/pod-product-compliance
Lightning Source LLC
Chambersburg PA
CBHW071411180526
45170CB00001B/71